BEATING BREAST CANCER

Life-saving choices
for South African women

John & Jenny Ireland

1993
Oxford
Cape Town

Oxford University Press
Walton Street, Oxford OX2 6DP, United Kingdom

Oxford New York Toronto
Delhi Bombay Calcutta Madras Karachi
Kuala Lumpur Singapore Hong Kong Tokyo
Nairobi Dar es Salaam Cape Town
Melbourne Auckland Madrid

and associated companies in
Berlin Ibadan

OXFORD is a trade mark of Oxford University Press

BEATING BREAST CANCER
ISBN 0 19 570869 5

© John Ireland 1993

Medical illustrations and flow charts: Fiona Calder
Illustrations: Michael Souter
Indexer: Sandy Vahl
Cover artwork: Michael Souter

Published by Oxford University Press Southern Africa,
Harrington House, Barrack Street, Cape Town 8001, South Africa

Set in 9$^{1}/_{2}$ pt on 12 pt Stone Serif by Theiner Typesetting (Pty) Ltd
Reproduction by Theiner Typesetting (Pty) Ltd
Cover reproduction by Fairstep
Printed and bound by Creda

Foreword

Congratulations to John and Jenny for converting the frightening problem of dealing with breast cancer into a positive experience. Many patients and their families comment that they only start real living after the diagnosis of breast cancer. Every day becomes a time to be enjoyed and appreciated, family and friends become more valuable, and each experience a treasured memory. The time prior to the diagnosis was grey, rushed, and stressed. The priorities of family and friends were secondary to the needs of work and money.

We all need information to help us convert the event of breast cancer from a hopeless and helpless experience to one of insight and planning. Information transforms us from passive puppets to active consumers, demanding our rights and making management decisions. The helpless, hopeless feelings are supplanted by an attitude of calm and control; chaos and fear are replaced by serenity. Once we are in control, however horrendous the position, we can cope.

I sometimes wonder whether doctors and nurses realize how much confusion we cause in our well-meaning attempts to explain an illness and alternative treatment options to patients. We try to sound competent and scientific, using medical jargon. Meanwhile the patient is frightened and confused, having difficulty concentrating, let alone understanding sophisticated medical terms.

Beating Breast Cancer is an excellent review of all aspects of breast cancer, including normal breast conditions. The emphasis is on accurate information presented clearly in words and diagrams. It is written in a warm, friendly, and encouraging manner, and John and Jenny encourage family participation in all aspects of breast disease. What a delight to have a book on breast cancer with a chapter for men — so often the forgotten factor in the breast equation.

I would like to see a copy of this book under the arm of every patient who visits her doctor about a breast problem. It will empower her and enable her to meet her medical team as an equal, with the confidence to share in decision-making.

Doctor Anne Hacking, Radiation Oncologist
Former Head of The Breast Cancer Clinic
Groote Schuur Hospital, Cape Town

Preface

People often do not want to hear, talk, or even read about cancer. I sincerely wish there were no need for a book such as this, but unfortunately there is. Most women are destined to have a breast lump, and therefore will have to face what it could mean, and decide what to do about it. Between one in nine and one in twelve westen women (depending on race and geographical location) will at some stage of their lives develop breast cancer. This is a sobering statistic indeed. By talking, reading, and generally being better informed about breast cancer, we can minimize the risks to ourselves and those close to us. We will also be better able to help and support women friends, partners, relatives, or colleagues for whom breast cancer becomes a real rather than a potential threat.

This book gives the salient facts regarding function of the breast, risk factors, early detection, management and surgical options, emotional responses and reactions, as well as common-sense advice. The book's aim is to inform and enlighten rather than frighten. Practical and philosophical personal attitudes are considered, with an emphasis on positive aspects and preventive action. Strategies are offered to help cope with the devastating diagnosis of cancer of the breast.

Men's role in helping women to deal with breast cancer is often overlooked, yet it is an essential ingredient of the overall coping and healing strategy, both from a physical and a mental point of view.

Fears and fallacies are realistically dealt with, as are the various options available.

Dedication

To my wife Jenny, whose example shines as a bright light to all; who epitomizes courage and positive thinking, and demonstrates the importance of having a practical, realistic approach to life.

Contents

Chapter 1

Choices

Introduction

Life involves a series of choices. These choices bring about certain results, often as expected, but sometimes unforeseen. We are the captains of our own ships in life and can steer our own course, but in uncharted seas the guidance of an experienced navigator is invaluable. So, too, can constructive guidance be invaluable when we are unsure of what course to take in life. I hope this book will be helpful in this regard.

The importance of decision-making is outlined in Figure 1.1, below. The rewards of deciding to choose, and then in turn of making choices which result in positive, affirmative action, are highlighted. The outcome is a sense of satisfaction and achievement.

Such a rewarding, decision-making course of action epitomizes the positive attitude also shown in the statement: 'I will overcome this hurdle in my life of a breast lump or cancer by doing and accepting that which is necessary'.

Being able to make the correct choices requires sufficient knowledge to weigh the pros and cons and thereby come to a logical, if sometimes painful, decision. Subsequent choices will be governed by developments. The aim of this book is to make you aware of the need to choose and the importance of doing so; to provide the information about breast cancer to enable such choices to be made on a balance of the facts; and to help with the further strategy of coping with the outcome and results of such decisions. This book addresses many aspects of breast cancer: increased awareness, insight, reasons, coping strategies, variables, and consequences. It considers what should, can, or must be done under different circumstances. Some of the choices involved are demanding in the extreme, and will be emotionally draining, but are necessary nevertheless. At the same time, emphasis is always placed on what there is to gain rather than on what there is to lose.

The process of learning

It has often been said that one is never too old to learn. While this is clearly correct, it is also strongly influenced by attitude and the willingness or need to learn. When being taught, it is irritating to be dictated or lectured to with little regard for your own thoughts or opinions on a particular subject. Under ideal circumstances a process of give-and-take should occur, with active, two-way participation between teacher and student.

With a book, this process is not easily achieved, as it provides a point of view without allowing for further discussion. As a reader, therefore, you have to assess the information and then accept or discard any advice given, as you see fit.

The process of teaching

After learning, the next step is often the process of teaching to others that which you yourself have learnt. I would like to suggest that if you gain something from this book, no matter how little, you please tell others about it. This passing-on of information is called the domino effect. Only by having many successive dominos will the information be spread to lots of people. So become a domino yourself — create an ongoing link, and for someone, sometime, somewhere you may save a lot of anguish. Together we can all inform a lot of people about the importance of taking positive action against breast cancer.

Declaring war on cancer

The word cancer strikes fear into all hearts. It is often the unseen and initially silent enemy which will strike when least expected. But in the case of breast cancer this foe can be detected early and can often be beaten. Cancer of the breast is the most common form of the disease in women, but is fortunately the one most easily detected in its early stages. The importance of an aggressive approach to early detection and treatment cannot be overstressed. The eradication of breast cancer has many stages, all requiring planning and appropriate strategy.

Stage one: Awareness and acceptance of breast cancer as a risk which requires defensive action and early detection. The risk increases with age, and so too must awareness. There are

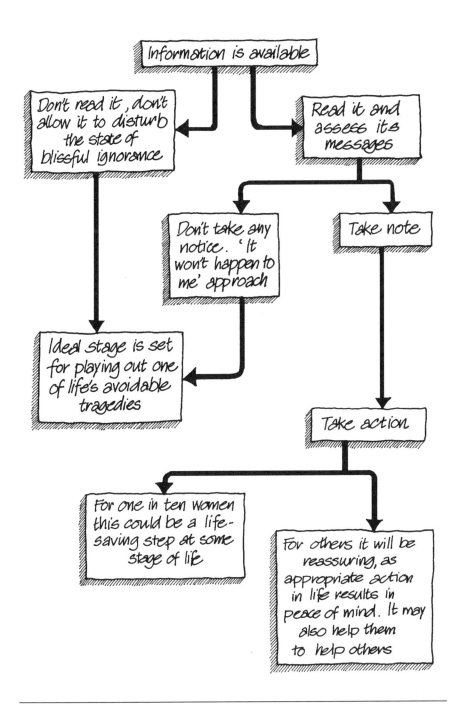

Figure 1.1 *This book is about choices*

different strategies employed in detection at different ages (see Chapter 4).

Stage two: If you detect a lump, seek medical attention immediately so as to determine whether or not it is cancer and then to get rid of it by mastectomy (removal of the breast) or lumpectomy (removal of the growth only).

Stage three: Further eradication of possible remaining cancer cells by using cytotoxics (chemotherapy) or irradiation.

Stage four: Recovering from the physical and emotional damage sustained during stages two and three.

Stage five: Adjusting to an uneasy truce whilst always on the alert for signs of further cancer developing. This may require further tests, follow-up, X-rays, scans, etc.

Stage six: Returning to a more peaceful situation but remaining watchful to avoid being caught unawares in the future.

Remaining neutral
does not work
in the war against cancer.

Supportive infrastructure

The man's role

During each of these six stages a woman will need male support, love, and understanding. In any woman's life there will be a male who can lend support — whether he be husband or lover, father, friend, son, or brother. Such males are an essential and irreplaceable part of the whole process of dealing with breast cancer, from detection through diagnosis, treatment, and then the phases of recovery.

The importance of a man's role is often minimized. The crucial part that men could, or should, play is often overlooked by men and women alike. Problems in relationships are then often created rather than solved, and aggravated rather than soothed. Such problems usually stem from underlying anxiety and anger as well as from fear and frustration. They are aggravated by 'silence', lack of understanding, and poor communication between a woman with breast cancer and the man or men in her life as regards hidden fears and emotions. Problems which remain in a state of ferment 'blow up' later unless the pressure can be released.

Discussion is the safety valve. An awareness of the man's role, with positive participation by him during the many different stages of intervention and decision-making, will be of major benefit. In most cases his help and encouragement, 'togetherness', mutual

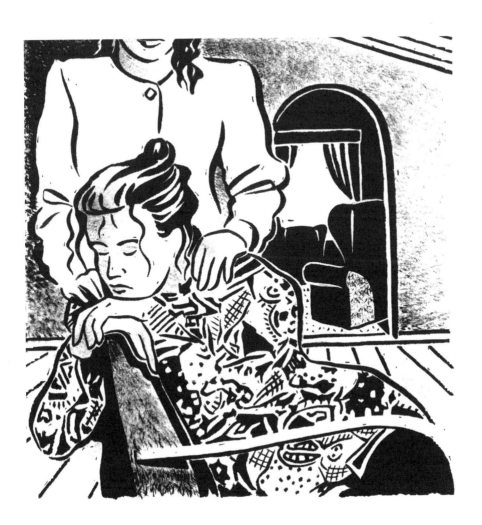

support, and understanding will allow an uncomplicated healing process to proceed. The man's role is as important as stitches or clips can be in helping a major wound to heal: healing can take place without them, but will almost certainly take longer and will leave an ugly, disfiguring scar. With breast cancer there will always be a scar, but it need not be physically, spiritually, or emotionally disfiguring.

Faced with a woman relative, friend, or lover with breast cancer, a man is often uncertain of his exact role, and may well withdraw because he is not sure what is expected of him. If his initial 'timid', supportive approaches are accepted and encouraged, he will continue to mature in his supportive role. If, however, his 'wanting to help but not knowing how' approach is initially rejected, for whatever reason, he will then tend to withdraw and isolate himself. Men's roles are discussed more extensively in Chapter 11.

Other supportive roles

The need for support varies tremendously from one person to another. Some prefer to keep to themselves, making their own plans and decisions, while others talk about their innermost fears and apprehensions and take advice readily. At some stage even the strongest women will need some form of support and guidance.

For those fortunate enough to have close family — husband, mother, father, brother, or sister — available, these people are often the most suitable source of help. For older women, a grown-up son or daughter can fulfil this need. For others without close family nearby, a good friend or minister of religion must then take the primary supportive role. Some women may need help from medical or psychiatric counsellors or professionals trained to guide patients through the bewildering and frightening paths of decision-making and acceptance (see Appendix for details).

Supportive roles are discussed more fully in Chapter 11.

We all have roles to play.

66 *When I was diagnosed as having breast cancer I could not change that fact, but I could choose how I would handle it, and I could choose my treatment options.* **Jenny** **99**

Chapter 2

Cancer and cell function

Cell structure and function

Each organ is comprised of millions of cells. Despite the different functions of the organs, all cells work using the same basic functions and principles (see Figure 2.1). The cell wall, or *membrane*, allows specific substances to pass through it in one or other direction at certain times, and thereby controls the make-up of the cell's contents (the *cytoplasm*). Within the cytoplasm are energy-providing units called *mitochondria*. There are also digestive vacuoles in the cell, called *lysosomes*. 'Food' for the lysosomes is prepared by the *golgi apparatus*.

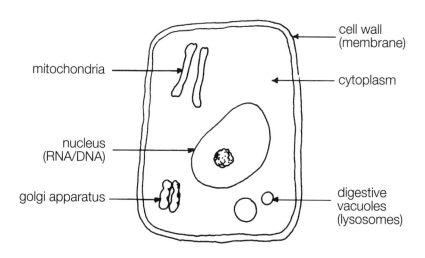

Figure 2.1 *Basic cell structure*

The *nucleus* is the cell's management centre. It contains chromo-somes comprised of deoxyribonucleic acid (DNA). These chromo-somes are duplicated exactly in every cell of that individual's body as the cells multiply. They are the genes which determine the species. The nucleus also contains ribonucleic acid (RNA), making up the ribosomes. The ribosomes produce certain types of protein which result in the specific function of that particular cell.

RNA is therefore responsible for making you an individual of a species which is determined by DNA. DNA determines *what* you are; RNA *who* you are. Multiplication of these normal cells is usually under strict and structured bodily control, and proceeds in a pre-determined and limited manner.

In much the same way that bricks can be used to build struc-tures that vary vastly in shape, size, and function, the body cells make up an enormous variety of organs, even though the principles governing the functioning of all body cells are essentially the same.

Normal cells compared to cancer cells

Normal cells are very much like cars. They burn up substances (fuel) to produce energy. They also produce waste products (equivalent to exhaust fumes) which must be got rid of (excreted). Cells come in many shapes and sizes, some slow and some fast, some young and some old. As they age and become decrepit, cells have to be replaced by new, active ones. Old ones are broken down by the body and their components either reused or excreted. Cells are usually arranged in a very structured way within each organ, like cars parked in a car park. As long as they all behave, there is a sense of order, and no damage occurs to neighbouring cars or surrounding struc-tures.

Cancer cells are like hot-rods driven by delinquents. They are different in shape and form. They have no respect for other cars. They bash and crash, and having wrecked one area, they move on to another. Their behaviour is erratic and unpredictable. They follow no set route, and may stay in one area for a while or leave without warning. They take over as the other meeker cars give way or are destroyed. The only way to destroy them, in turn, is to physically remove them and tow them away (surgery) or to destroy their engines (irradiation) or fuel/energy system (cytotoxics/chemother-apy).

The body's immune system functions much like a traffic-police force attempting to track down and control the hot-rods that escape. The immune system cannot, however, control cancer cells once

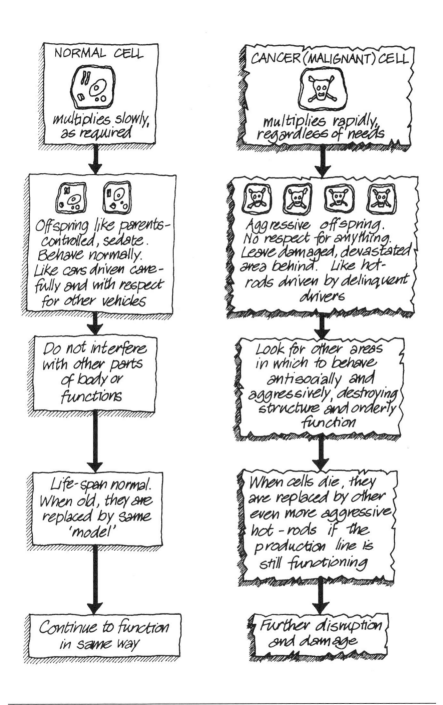

Figure 2.2 *Comparison of behaviour of normal cells and cancer cells*

there are too many of them. The quality of the immune system — the officers in the traffic-police force — also varies from one individual to another and from time to time. It is affected by illness and by nutrition and stress. It can usually cope with individual hot-rods (early cancer-cell detection and destruction), but cannot cope with the whole gang (established cancer); it then needs help in the form of surgery, irradiation, and cytotoxic drugs.

> *Cancers are cells out of control.*
> *There are ways to control them.*

What is cancer?

My daughter once said, 'It is the word cancer that kills.' The word cancer is derived from the Latin meaning 'crab'. The word cancer also means any dangerous and spreading evil — presumably linked to early concepts of the crab's shape and movement.

What types of cancer are there?

There are many types of cancer which can occur in or arise from the many different types of tissue cells throughout the body. Each cell type gives rise to its own kind of cancer, with its own causes, frequency, symptoms, treatment, and outcomes. Some cancers are more common than others; some are more dangerous; some are more responsive to certain forms of treatment; some are more rapid-growing and invasive, while others are more localized. The one common denominator is that when any normal cell becomes a cancer cell it undergoes a dangerous change, especially as regards its behaviour pattern. It becomes a 'rogue cell', which loses all respect for a structured, peaceful co-existence with other cells. The fundamental change is one of uncontrolled cellular multiplication. Cancer cells overwhelm, destroy, and replace normal cells. The body is, however, not entirely defenceless, and can recognize and destroy cancer cells through different immune mechanisms which are discussed later in this chapter.

What is a tumour?

The word *tumour* merely means a growth. Tumours are in turn classified as benign or malignant. The term *benign* means the tumour is non-invasive, and that although there is an overgrowth of cells locally, the only problem these cells cause is one of obstruction or compression of surrounding tissue. Benign tumours do not invade or replace other tissue, as is the case with cancer-cell invasion. Benign tumours can usually be removed without further problems.

What does malignant mean?

The term *malignant* is used for those tumours which do not have a 'fence' or 'capsule' around them. Malignant tumours invade (cancer), and destroy the function of the host tissue in which they occur. They tend to spread, either directly (*local invasion*) or to other parts of the body via the blood or lymph systems. The malignant cells continue to invade the organs they find themselves in. The *lesions* away from the original site are called *secondaries* or *metastases*.

What are the implications of secondaries?

The sites of secondary spread are often preferred by certain types of cancer. They commonly include local glands, skin, lung, liver, bone or brain. Once spread has occurred it is much more difficult both to detect and to destroy the cancer. Treatment under such circumstances is therefore altered accordingly. During broader and more aggressive treatment regimes other innocent cells are unavoidably damaged. Hair and bone marrow are typical examples of such innocent bystanders that suffer in the fight against cancer cells.

The reason why hair and bone marrow are affected by cytotoxic treatment (drugs administered to kill cancer cells) is because they consist of rapidly-dividing cells (making new hair and new blood cells) which are more sensitive to damage than other slower-growing cells in the body (see the section on Cytotoxics/chemotherapy in Chapter 9). Such hair loss (it does regrow) or bone marrow suppression is the price paid during this phase of treatment. The suppression of bone marrow has to be carefully monitored with blood tests.

Where do breast cancers spread to?

The first spread tends to be to skin or to local lymph glands in the armpit (axillary) or behind the breastbone (sternal). Thereafter breast cancers tend to spread to lungs, liver, bone, or brain.

What types of cancer occur in the female breast?

Cancer in situ: Ductal or lobular

The words *in situ* mean that the cancer is still contained within the area in which it started and that it has not invaded other tissue, even locally. In the breast, cancer *in situ* can either be within the ducts or in the lobules (breast glandular tissue). Lobular carcinoma *in situ* will only become invasive in about 30% of women. Ductal carcinoma *in situ*, on the other hand, is much more likely to become invasive at some stage.

Invasive carcinoma: Ductal or lobular

The word invasive indicates that the cancer is no longer contained within the duct or lobule where it originated and that it has infiltrated (spread to) surrounding tissue.

Other forms

There are other uncommon histological types of cancer which occur in only a small percentage of patients and will therefore not be mentioned here.

Can men get breast cancer?

Yes, men can get breast cancer, but it is very uncommon. For every hundred women with breast cancer there will be less than one case occurring in a man.

Men	Women
Skin	Skin
Lung	Breast
Prostate	Uterus/cervix
Large bowel (colon)	Large bowel (colon)

Children

Cancers common in children differ from those in adults and tend to affect the glands (lymphatic tissue, therefore called lymphomas), marrow (leukaemia), kidney, brain, and bone.

Table 2.1 *Common cancers*

What are the characteristics of all cancers?

There are over a hundred different types of cancer that can occur in humans. Characteristics common to all types are:

Stage 1: Uncontrolled growth which starts in a single cell
Stage 2: Localization as a mass
Stage 3: Invasion of local tissues
Stage 4: Metastasis (spread) to other parts of the body via bloodstream or lymph system, or both

All cancers go through these stages. The rate at which they do so varies with the type of cancer and from one individual to another.

Development of breast cancer

What factors play a role?

As breast cancer (after skin cancer) is the most common cancer in European and North American women, much has been done to try to determine which factors influence its development. It is projected that by the year 2000 there will be over 1.2 million new cases of breast cancer per year throughout the world. What must be remembered is that symptomatic cancer is the end stage of a sequence of cell changes and events that have usually taken place over years. We all at times produce cancer cells in our bodies, but only some of us will ever develop cancer. The reasons for this are still poorly understood. Statistically some of the following factors are important, but it must be stressed not necessarily so in a particular individual.

Who is at risk?

General summary of influencing factors:
- increased risk after the age of thirty; levels out for women in their 40s, and increases again thereafter;
- increased risk in Western European and American women as compared with Asian, African, and Japanese women;
- increased incidence in upper social classes;
- increased incidence in unmarried women over 40;
- increased risk in women who have never breast-fed;
- risk two to three times higher if either parent had breast cancer; five times higher if both mother and sister had breast cancer;
- increased incidence in obese women;
- increased incidence if exposed to radiation;

- increased incidence in women who have had another cancer of ovary, uterus, or large bowel;
- possible increased risk after events involving severe emotional stress;
- recently an increasing incidence in younger women (under 35 years).

The role of race

This is a complex factor. The incidence of breast cancer in North America and Western Europe is six to ten times greater than in Japan, most parts of Asia, and Africa. While a genetic disposition or protection factor may play a role, so do many other factors such as breast-feeding practices, diet, size of families, degrees of stress, and forms of contraception. In addition, the incidence of breast cancer in people with traditionally low rates changes when they move to a higher-risk country and adopt the life-style of that country.

The role of hormones

While female hormones undoubtedly play a role, exactly how normal hormonal changes promote or affect breast-cancer development is still not understood. Oestrogen undoubtedly promotes the growth of some forms of breast cancer, and therefore post-menopausal hormone-replacement therapy (HRT) is not advisable for women who have had breast cancer.

As regards the contraceptive pill, some studies have shown that starting to use it at an early age and then using it for a long time does lead to increased risk. However, other studies appear to contradict this.

Nutrition

High-fat diets: Once again there have been contradictory findings: in laboratory rats there is a clear increase of breast cancer in rats fed a high-fat diet and which are then given a cancer-causing product (carcinogen). Looking at migrant workers, for example Japanese women in the USA, it would seem that high-fat diets early on in life are much more important. The incidence of breast cancer increases only in Japanese girls born and raised in the USA, and not in Japanese women moving to the USA as adults who only then change to a high-fat diet.

Sugar: High sugar intake has been linked to an increased likelihood of breast cancer. The reasons for this are unclear.

Other factors: Even the drinking of alcohol has been linked to increased risk of breast cancer, but to separate its effect from the other dietary factors is very difficult.

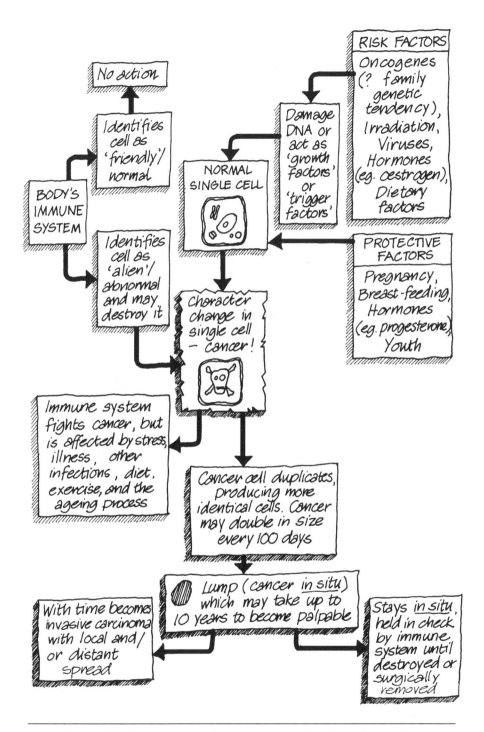

Figure 2.3 *Development of breast cancer: Possible influential factors*

Over-nutrition in post-menopausal women, who are consequently obese, has been linked with higher oestrogen levels and also with an increased incidence of breast cancer.

Cancer genes

These are called *oncogenes*, and we all have them — luckily usually in a dormant form. Exactly what 'wakes them up' and sets them off is unclear. It may be the natural ageing process of our body (cancer incidence increases markedly with ageing), or a specific viral infection (there is some evidence for this), or other factors such as stress which are as yet unconfirmed.

Our own immune system is very important in recognizing these oncogenes as enemies and then destroying or controlling them when they become active. Changes with age which affect this immune-system recognition and response may therefore be important.

Radiation

We are all exposed to radiation. It is usually low-level radiation such as that which occurs with television, computer screens, digital watches, clocks, and radios. Higher exposure is usually as a result of X-ray investigations. People exposed to very high-energy, ionizing radiation, such as when atomic explosions or accidents occur, suffer an increased incidence of breast cancer as well as of other cancers. This is due to the genetic structure of the cells (DNA) being damaged by the irradiation.

There is also an increased risk of developing cancer in tissues which are exposed to radiation while it is being used to treat (destroy) cancer in a certain area. This is termed the 'edge effect' or 'fringe effect' and occurs in cells damaged by radiation but not killed. Such cells and their offspring show an increased tendency to malignant change with time. This is a factor that must be borne in mind by younger women who choose lumpectomy with radiation: long-term changes in the underlying lung or remaining breast tissue may become a potential problem. While it is clear that low-energy sun radiation does cause skin cancer from over-exposure, there is little evidence that exposure to the sun's radiation influences breast cancer at all.

Age

None of us can avoid ageing. While cancer incidence increases with age, this may well be because cancer can take years to develop. In other words, the cancer-causing changes start when we are much younger. However, our immune protection may not be as effective

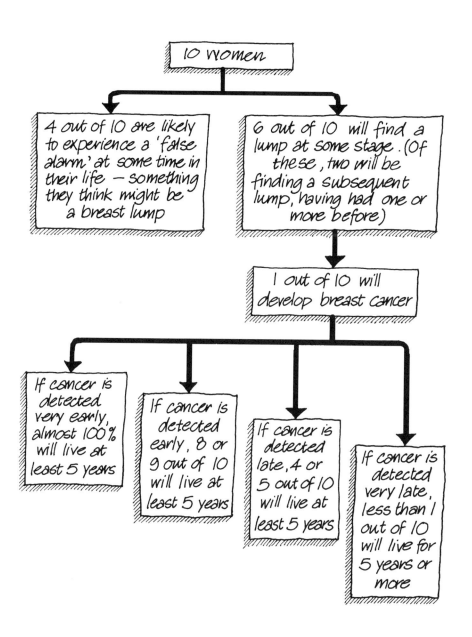

Figure 2.4 *You are not alone*

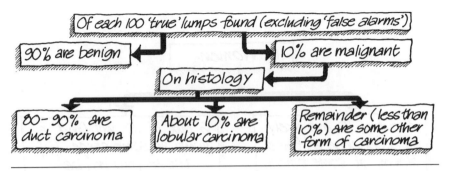

Figure 2.5 *Not all lumps are malignant*

in protecting us from our own cancer cells as we grow older, enabling cancer to get the upper hand as we age.

Stress

There may be a connection between severe emotional stress, such as bereavement or divorce, and subsequent cancer progression. Stress undoubtedly effects our immune system (body defence mechanisms), and it is probably this that reduces our ability to hold potential cancer cells in check, and thus leads to progression. Stress-coping skills are therefore important not only in the stressful situations we face in everyday life, but also in the way we handle the diagnosis and treatment of cancer itself.

Cancer which was probably there all along, but was being effectively controlled by the body's defence system, advances following stress as our defences are weakened during this vulnerable stage.

What to do about risk factors

With so many factors being incriminated we clearly cannot select any one to hold responsible for the development of breast cancer. Each factor should not be seen in isolation, so do not worry because you think you fall into a particular category. However, it is important to recognize that some or all of these factors increase the risk of breast cancer. The ones that we have control over are those that can be changed or modified (such as diet and how we handle stress). The other factors we can ignore, as there is little point in worrying about something you cannot change.

Accepting the things that cannot be changed requires mature insight and is often easier said than done. Bear in mind that most things in life done in moderation are unlikely to be harmful, so change need not always be drastic.

66 *There are no guarantees in life.* **John** **99**

Chapter 3

The breast itself

How important is the breast in society?

The act of feeding (suckling) our young on milk secreted from mammary glands in the breast is what makes us mammals (as compared with fish, birds, or reptiles). Breasts are by nature designed as purely functional feeding organs, which in primitive societies were not considered as anything more than this. Throughout most of known history, however, the breast has become the established symbol of womanhood. It has been covered or exposed to greater or lesser extents depending on accepted norms and fashions for particular periods or societies. Breasts do represent much more in our lives than merely a source of sustenance for babies.

During the 1960s and 70s, ardent advocates of feminism tried to oust the breast from its representative role as the ultimate symbol of femininity. But the 'burn the bra' stage was short-lived and generally unsuccessful. The breast has been, and probably always will be, a symbol of femininity. It plays a part in sexual stimulation and arousal, and therefore has sexual connotations too. From early childhood, exposure to the importance and 'role' of breasts is inescapable in conversation, attitudes, jokes, video and TV, and everyday advertising of bathing costumes and other fashions.

We would be bluffing ourselves if we imagined a society where the breast would represent only a feeding function, and where it was unimportant to men. Many woman find it demeaning (and quite rightly so) when attention is paid to what they are endowed with rather than who they are. Women with small breasts are sometimes made to feel inferior; others with very large breasts are embarrassed by gawkish looks and crude or even so-called 'complimentary' comments. Others display and exploit their breasts to achieve as much effect on the opposite sex as possible. For women with different cultural and ethnic backgrounds, outlooks, morals, and upbringing, breasts represent many different things. I doubt that they are ever truly unimportant, even for those who claim indifference. Many women are very conscious of their femininity, take pleasure in their sexuality, and certainly consider their breasts an integral part of their whole living process.

The image of catastrophic disfigurement through the loss of a breast is often what is most feared as the inevitable consequence of having breast cancer. Ask a woman what she dreads most and many will answer 'breast cancer'. Yet what is actually meant in the majority of cases is 'losing a breast'. The reality of what breast cancer could mean as regards life and health usually comes later. First thoughts are about disfigurement, loss of femininity, loss of sexuality, and are certainly not that mastectomy may be a life-saving procedure and in a bizarre way something to be 'thankful' for. That femininity and sexuality *need not be lost* is not seen in perspective initially, and their loss is assumed to be an inevitable consequence of mastectomy.

The very word mastectomy tends to strike fear into the bravest of hearts. Such fears often hinder timely diagnosis and result in delay in seeking help and treatment. Losing a breast is damaging to mind, body, and emotions. Adjusting to it happening will require courage and willpower, and positive logical thinking of the highest order.

Femininity is largely a state of mind and attitude, and the loss of a breast need not alter this either for a woman or for the men in her life. Logic and emotion are often contradictory: how can the loss of a breast ever be compared to the gaining of a life which is so often the direct result? Certainly it is a loss of major proportions, and adapting to it will be difficult. But if viewed in a mature, reflective way, regaining a life — and with it a new, more caring value system — is an enormous asset.

Normal structure and function of the breast

Newborns

In the newborn baby, the dormant breast tissue may have been stimulated by maternal and placental feminizing hormones and therefore may be enlarged (*gynaecomastica*) or even secrete milk! This effect is short-lived, and the breasts return to 'normal' without treatment. Parents should be informed so that they understand it is only a side-effect of maternal hormonal action.

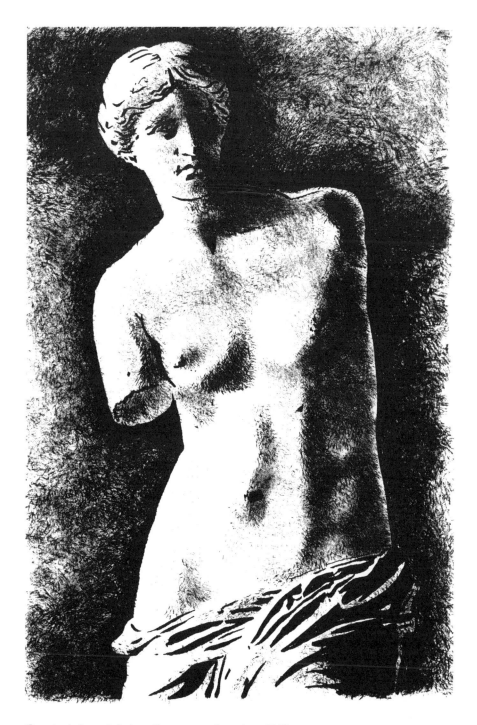

Greek statue of Aphrodite, second century B.C.

Puberty

Throughout childhood a girl's breast remains dormant (quiescent), awaiting the stimulation of increased feminizing hormones at puberty. About three years before actual menstruation starts, the breast tissue under the nipple and areola (darker pigmented area around the nipple) starts developing. This onset of breast development is called the *thelarche*. The onset of menstruation is called the *menarche*. Breasts are not fully developed until regular menstrual cycles with ovulation (egg production by the ovaries) occur. The onset of hair growth in the armpits (*axillae*) and pubic area is called the *pubarche*, and usually accompanies the other changes. If these changes start in a very young child (less than eight years old) it is then called *precocious puberty* and must be investigated, as some of the potential causes are serious.

How does this all come about?

There is a complex interaction through hormones and feedback mechanism between specific areas of the brain (the hypothalamus and pituitary gland) and the ovaries. The hypothalamus and pituitary gland stimulate and regulate hormone release, and the hormones in turn affect specific target organs. The development of the female secondary sex characteristics (in body shape and breast function) is dependent on the presence and interaction of many hormones as well as on the absence of male (androgen and testosterone) hormones. The *synergistic* action (working together) of the female hormones (*oestrogen* and *progesterone*), messengers to the organs (*gonadotrophins*), and growth hormone from the pituitary gland are all part of the complex process of becoming an adult female.

How do hormones work?

Hormones are powerful substances produced by different glands at different times and in varying amounts (often very small) in the body. They act as messengers to cells in other parts of the body, telling them how and when to do something specific. There are also complex interactions between hormones, and feedback mechanisms to 'switch off' the messenger once a sufficient quantity of a product has been produced, or enough action taken. Hormones 'tell' breast tissue when to develop and when to stop developing. On a monthly basis hormones cause the breasts to prepare for a possible pregnancy; and when the hormone levels fall (no pregnancy) the breast returns to normal. If pregnancy does occur, ongoing hormonal stimulation causes further glandular tissue to develop and milk production to occur.

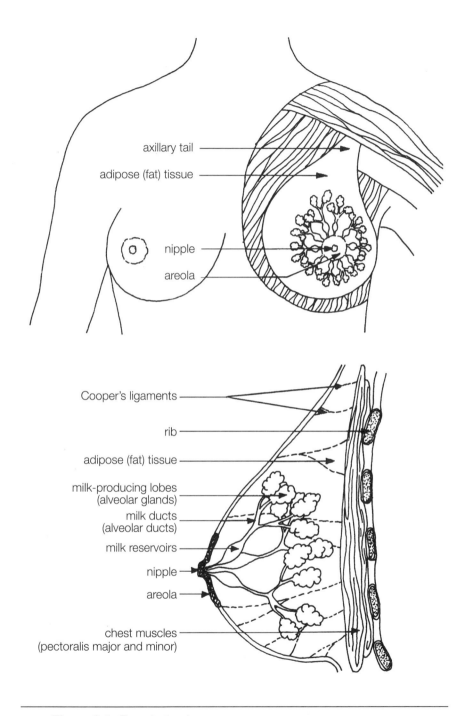

Figure 3.1 *Breast structure*

The breasts of a woman who is not pregnant consist mainly of fat (two-thirds of the volume), with actual breast tissue (secretory lobules) making up one-third. In pregnancy, with the simultaneous action of female hormones (oestrogen and progesterone), *prolactin* (milk-stimulating hormone), thyroid and growth hormones, the breast changes markedly, and by the end of pregnancy consists almost entirely of secretory (milk-producing) lobules. The production of milk is called *lactation*, with prolactin being the main milk-stimulating hormone (see Figure 3.2). As well as producing milk, breasts are also effective and sterile packaging for the product.

Menstruation

The menstrual cycle occurs in anticipation of a possible pregnancy. Each month the uterus is prepared to receive the fertilized ovum, and if this does not occur, normal menstruation takes place. During the menstrual cycle there are changes in hormonal levels which affect the breasts. In some women, during the second half of the cycle their breasts become nodular and tender. If such breast tenderness is severe it is called *mastalgia*. The main hormone causing this change is probably progesterone.

This recurring nodularity of the breast can be confused with lumps caused by growths, so examination of the breast should be done once menstruation has occurred, i.e., during the first half of the cycle. Any nodule 'lump' found during the second half of a menstrual cycle must be reassessed immediately after the cycle is over. If it is still present it should be investigated (see Chapter 4).

Other conditions affecting the breast

Like other organs in the body, breasts can be affected by many different conditions. First, and most importantly, **most lumps found are benign**. So don't panic if you find one. It may be a cyst, a benign fat tumour (*lipoma*), fibrous disease, fat necrosis (usually after local trauma and injury to breast tissue), a duct papilloma (benign duct tumour), or fibrocytic disease of the breast. I can almost hear you saying, 'It's all very well for him to say don't panic!', but it is important to keep the risk factors in perspective. You will be bound to worry about finding a lump, but try not to panic about it.

If there is associated pain, tenderness, and inflammation, then an abscess, infected cyst, or mastitis is likely to be the underlying cause.

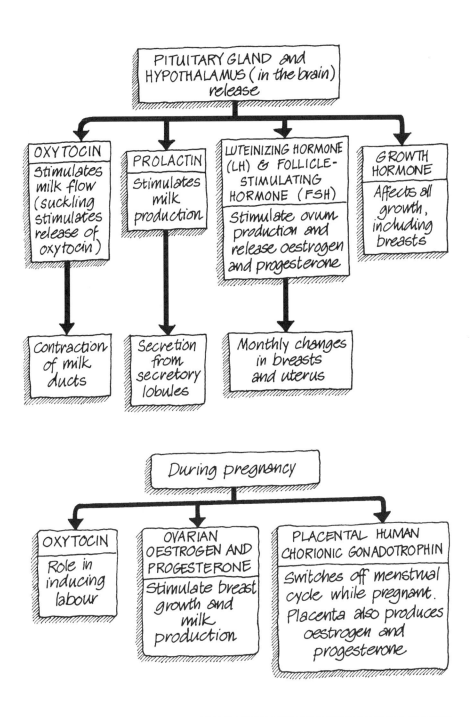

Figure 3.2 *Main hormonal pathways*

The skin of the breast and nipple can become irritated and chafed (for example in 'jogger's nipples'), or may be affected by contact with clothing, soaps, and detergents that cause local dermatitis or eczema. These conditions can mimic Paget's Disease of the nipple, which is associated with an underlying cancer of the breast, so further investigation must be done to ascertain whether such nipple conditions are a risk.

In some women, a non-bloody nipple discharge such as is quite common during pregnancy may occur with normal monthly hormonal cyclical changes. Other benign intraductal pathology such as papillomas can also cause a nipple discharge. If the discharge is a new event, however, associated with a lump, skin disorder, or nipple retraction, or is bloody, then an immediate medical consultation must be arranged. Do not wait to see if it will go away by itself. Take precautions — see a doctor!

66 *I never felt any the less feminine or attractive after my mastectomy. I believe a woman's sensuality is in her eyes, her smile, and most of all her heart.* **Jenny**   **99**

Chapter 4

Detection

Introduction: Your life is in your own hands

In many ways each of us can exert a major influence over our own life. Some of us have major drawbacks and difficulties to overcome, others have virtually none, but we can affect almost every aspect to a greater or lesser extent. One aspect that we all hope and pray for is that we will be blessed with good health. So what can we do about health? Actually a lot. Through the way we live, work, eat, drink, and play we can either improve or damage our health. Many of these important aspects of our life-style are covered elsewhere in the book (Chapters 9 and 11). In addition, we must be aware of the need to take preventive action — or at the very least ensure early detection of conditions which could shorten our potential lifespan. Cancers in particular demand early detection, and cancer of the breast is among the most accessible in this regard. Successful results can often be obtained with the implementation of prompt treatment following such early detection. With the current trend being towards breast-preserving procedures, there is even greater motivation for breast self-examination (BSE). There is so much to be gained from early detection.

Self-examination: The pros and cons

Background

Self-examination for breast cancer is an important preventive procedure. Initially it was strongly supported by health practitioners, but it appears that it is being unceremoniously 'dumped' by some authorities. Recent newspaper headlines declared: 'Shock U-turn on DIY breast cancer checks'. Others claimed: 'There is no scientific evidence that self-examination helps to detect breast cancer early.

All it does is create a phobia and ongoing fear as regards what it might detect.'

I cannot for the life of me understand this attitude. A survey of any available statistics shows that cancer of the breast is discovered by the patient herself in 70–80% of cases. With the current increase in mammography, the proportion of lumps found by this new method of examination is increasing, but the majority of lumps are still found by the patient. This may be as a casual finding (large lump) or because of associated symptoms (skin dimpling/nipple discharge), by a partner during love-making, or through a routine self-examination.

If, as it is claimed, self-examination is not finding the lump early enough, then the fault lies not with the concept but with the way it is being done. Either the examination is being done in an unsystematic, superficial fashion to get it over with, or when something is found there is a delay in seeking medical help.

I found my wife's cancer during a routine breast examination when it was a mere 0.5 cm lump. I strongly believe that once women are fully informed about the importance of careful and meaningful self-examination, and once it becomes a routine in their lives without being cloaked in fear and apprehension, it can be extremely effective in the early detection of breast cancer.

Many of the authorities speaking out against self-examination advocate the routine use of mammography to replace clinical self-examination. I do not dispute the importance of mammography (see Chapter 4), but these two methods of examination compliment one another and should not be allowed to become mutually exclusive. Clearly there is a need for better education of women on the hows and whys of breast self-examination.

Know your own breasts

Examining you own breasts properly is not difficult. In fact, who knows your body and breasts better than you yourself. If their shape, texture, consistency, and nodularity are well-known to you through repeated examination, then you are well-placed to detect any changes early. Sometimes even doctors, who should set an example, do no more than a cursory 'scout' around the breasts when they examine them. This is to be deplored: a careful, systematic form of palpation should be demonstrated to all women, and they should be strongly advised and encouraged to carry out meaningful self-examination.

How and when should self-examination be done?

First, understand what the aim is: The aim is to detect as early as possible any change which could signify underlying cancer, and

Cancer creed: The power of positive thinking
I trust and pray I won't ever
get a lump and
especially not cancer but
if I do I must:
Find it (or have it found) early
and, when found, do something
about it immediately so that
If benign:
I can relax and get on with my life,
but I will keep on looking and remain vigilant.

If malignant:
I will
Be 'thankful' for finding it
Be 'grateful' that it was found early
Believe that I can be cured.

Remember that not finding
it would not mean
that it did not exist.
It is therefore better to find
it early, while something can and
will be done about it.

Be grateful for gains
rather than sad about losses.

thereby allow the widest choice of treatment and the best chance for a full and uncomplicated recovery.

■ Do it **regularly** and get to know your breasts. It only takes a few minutes each time.

■ Do it **routinely** after each menstrual cycle (period) ends.

■ If you are post-menopausal, do it on a **set day** each month.

When you do it, be systematic and careful (see Figure 4.1)

1 **Look** before you feel.
   a Stand in front of a mirror, with your arms at your sides, and look for any asymmetry (difference in shape between right and left breasts, which may of course always have been there), skin dimpling, or discharge from the nipple.

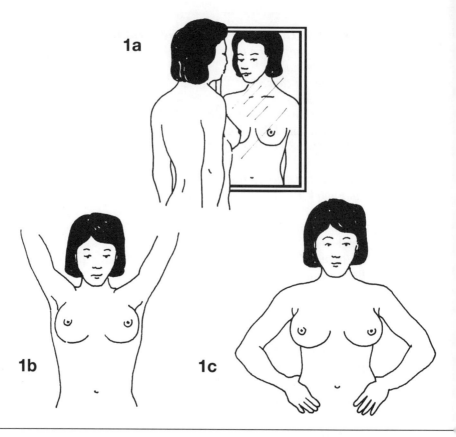

Figure 4.1 *Breast self-examination*

    b   Raise your arms above your head and turn from side to side, looking at your breasts from different angles.

    c   Place your hands on your hips and push inwards, thereby tensing the chest muscles.

2   After looking, you must palpate (feel) your breasts.

(Many women do not like touching or feeling their own breasts, and are self-conscious about it, but this is an attitude which can and must be overcome.)

    a   Squeeze your nipple gently between your fingers to see if there is any discharge.

    b   Now lie down on a bed. Place a small pillow or folded towel under one shoulder. Put that arm back up above and behind your head. This spreads the breast tissue out across the chest wall. Starting at the outer edge of the breast tissue, use your fingers to gently 'roll' the breast tissue against the chest

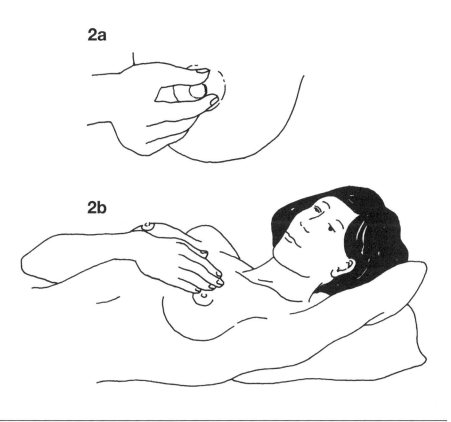

2a

2b

wall. This 'rolling' action is very important, as the small circular movements allow the breast tissue to move under the finger tips so that any local hardness or lump will be felt.

It must be stressed that normal breast-tissue lobules are nodular rather than fatty, and can be felt as such. So don't panic while getting to know your breasts. As you get used to the feel of them, so you will be more comfortable with what you are feeling, and you are then more likely to detect any change. Using this rolling technique, go round and round in ever-decreasing circles until the whole breast, including the tissue under the nipple area, has been carefully felt.

The breast also has an axillary tail (breast tissue which goes up into the armpit). Therefore place your fingers right up into the armpit and with the same 'rolling' motion against the chest wall feel the tissue (potential glands and breast tissue are in this area), working downwards carefully and steadily until you reach the edge of the breast tissue which you have already assessed.

c   Now repeat the procedure for the other breast.

d   If you have not felt anything out of the ordinary, you can relax, with peace of mind being the reward for a job well done. If, however, you find anything that worries you, phone a doctor straight away and make an appointment for a follow-up examination.

Self-examination must become routine, and although it will never be a comfortable experience, it need not be a frightening one. Breast examination does not prevent cancer occurring, but it does help you to detect it earlier should it start. This affects the prognosis (outlook or risk) and the nature, duration, and likely success of treatment.

You are the best person to examine your own breasts.

Examination by a doctor

If I have not been able to convince you that you should examine your breasts yourself, or if you find it too daunting and frightening or distasteful, then there are other ways to have your breasts examined. (It may be helpful at this stage to reread the section on Choices in Chapter 1).

One of the regular events in any woman's life should be a yearly visit to a gynaecologist or GP. One of the other common cancers specific to women is cancer of the cervix. While a vaginal examination and pap smear is regarded as an unpleasant experience for many women, it is important that it be done once a year. The doctor will examine your breasts at the same time. This serves the purpose of preventive examination, but breast examination should be done far more often than once a year.

As you get older (after the age of 50), breast and vaginal examination with a pap smear should be done twice a year due to the increased risks associated with ageing.

Mammography, ultrasonography, & thermography

The indications for these three methods of diagnostic investigation and their respective techniques, strengths, and weaknesses are considered and contrasted in this section.

Mammography

This is the specialized technique used for taking X-rays of the breasts (mammograms). X-rays of the breasts are not a new development, and were in fact first done more than 60 years ago. Techniques, equipment, and the amount of irradiation exposure have improved dramatically over the past 20 years, however, with the result that this form of investigation has now become a valuable and safe diagnostic tool. It still has its limitations and specific indications.

The amount of irradiation exposure during the procedure is now ten times less than it used to be. The RAD is the term used for a measure of radiation (much like volts for electricity, or metres for distance). Although a mammogram is an X-ray, and therefore must involve radiation, the amount of radiation that this investigation exposes you to is 0.1 to 0.2 of a RAD — a very small amount. So even if done on an annual basis, the risk of local tissue damage and subsequent breast-cancer development from the radiation involved is very small indeed. It has been estimated that only after 100 RADS of exposure does the incidence of breast cancer increase significantly, which would require at least 500 mammograms!

There are two main indications for mammograms:

1   Either assessment of a lump/mass found clinically by the patient or doctor, together with assessment of the other breast to help with diagnosis and with planning the nature of further treatment and management; or assessment of the breasts because of specific symptoms such as nipple discharge.

2   Screening programmes for the early detection of unsuspected cancer in a 'high-risk' (increased risk) group of asymptomatic patients. Higher risk can be because of:

  ■   age (over 50 years);
  ■   family history of breast cancer;
  ■   previous cancer in one breast;
  ■   underlying pre-cancerous breast disease; or
  ■   hormonal replacement therapy (HRT).

How is mammography done?   The technique involves the squeezing of the breast firmly between two surfaces to flatten it (this can be quite uncomfortable). X-rays are then taken through the flattened breast tissue in different directions — from top to bottom, side to side, and obliquely. Like any other X-ray examination, the technique relies on the fact that X-rays (which are invisible) will pass through tissue to greater or lesser extents depending on the density of that tissue. The receiving plate (like a photographic negative), then records the amount of rays reaching it and their varying strengths. The 'picture' therefore shows the density of the tissue that the rays have travelled through. A lesion such as cancer, with its increased density (which is why it is felt as a hard lump) will block off more rays and not allow them to pass through easily. It will therefore be seen on the X-ray plate as a white, dense lesion when compared with the surrounding breast tissue. Unfortunately breast tissue and other non-cancerous lesions in the breast can also vary in density.

It is thus clear that while the technique is very useful, it is not infallible. Other conditions cause increased density (including dense breast glandular tissue, as occurs in younger women and some older ones) which makes interpretation of mammograms more difficult. These conditions can camouflage the cancer which is present or mimic cancer where there is none.

Routine screening: Different authorities advise on different forms of screening programmes. Their efficacy for mass screening of women over the age of 50 is almost undisputed. When combined with regular clinical examination, screening done on an annual basis in the over-50 age group can reduce deaths from breast cancer by between 30 and 70%, according to various studies. This is an average reduction of 50%!

Indications for possible screening at a younger age (30–40 age group):
- family history of breast cancer;
- very early menarche (starting menstruation), long-term use of oral contraceptives, or first child born after 30 years of age;
- major fear about possible underlying breast cancer in a particular patient, where ordinary reassurance and clinical examination has not set her mind at rest. Such a patient may have lost a friend or relative from breast cancer.

Indications for annual screening at an older age:
- all women over the age of 50 have a higher risk;
- all women on hormonal replacement therapy over the age of 40.

Indications for screening asymptomatic women aged between 40 and 50: As risk in this age group is relatively small, it is recommended that a mammogram be done every two to three years.

Diagnostic indications: Any woman over the age of 30 with a palpable breast mass (lump) warrants a mammogram. This includes assessing the other breast. With routine, low-cost, screening mammography a single-view mammogram is often used, while a diagnostic mammogram will have two or three views of each breast, taken for a full and complete assessment.

Is this technique accurate and can it be depended on?
The answer is *no*. There may be up to a 10% or even 15% false negative rate. This means that 10–15% of cancerous lesions may not
show up on a mammogram. If your doctor is still worried about the
characteristics of the lump, even though the mammogram is negative, she may request an ultrasound examination or insist that you
have a biopsy (where a tiny piece of the lump is taken for analysis).
A biopsy is the safer path to follow, even though it may give you
sleepless nights until the histology result is available.

On the other hand, up to 7% false positive diagnoses may occur,
where the mammogram shows what looks like cancer but the lesion
is in fact benign. In the case of such a positive diagnosis, major
worry, followed by tremendous relief when the biopsy result is available, is a most traumatic experience to have to go through.

Mammograms are an important means of evaluating breast
masses (and other breast complaints) in women over the age of 30
(some authorities would say over 40). Below the age of 30, denser
normal breast tissue makes evaluation much less informative and
more difficult to interpret. Also, regular exposure to irradiation
when so young may prove to be dangerous when a woman is older.
The result of a mammogram is a guide to what further steps should
be taken, but the results are not entirely reliable.

Ultrasound

This is another non-invasive way of assessing the breast and the
masses/lumps within it. The principle is simple, and relies on non-
audible sound waves which are emitted from a transducer. These
waves travel through the different tissues and send back messages
about the size, shape, and consistency (density) of the tissue they are
passing through. These messages are transformed into a picture
which can be seen on a screen, much like a TV set. Ultrasound
examination requires skill and experience on the part of the operator for accurate interpretation of the sound-wave-pattern picture.

What are the advantages?

■ Painless, and less uncomfortable than a mammogram;

■ perhaps less embarrassing, depending on your point of view and
the operator;

■ extremely accurate (95–100%) in defining the difference between a solid mass and a cyst. If it is a cyst it can be aspirated
there and then under direct vision, and be seen to disappear
(collapse down). Cystic fluid, if bloody, will be sent for histology
(analysis). This aspiration of course then becomes an invasive
breast examination, but the service is offered by many of the
ultrasonographers and is extremely useful and accurate.

What are the disadvantages?

- Not as accurate in detecting cancerous masses with micro-calcification (a typical finding on mammogram in 40% of cancers);
- greater overlap between the sonographic (ultrasound) features of benign and malignant solid masses in the breast;
- not as accurate as mammography for consistently demonstrating small masses.

It must be stressed that the skill and experience of the operator can increase or lessen many of these potential disadvantages. Be guided by your doctor, and if she is happy with the particular ultrasound service then use it.

Thermography

I have included this just in case you have heard about it and wonder what it is. This technique has featured in a few magazines showing dramatic pictures of the mapping of the infrared output from cold and hot areas on the surface of the breast. While thermography is bright, colourful, and impressive, most authorities seem to agree that it is too inaccurate a technique for diagnosing breast cancer and is unreliable with current equipment. It should therefore be of interest but not relied on; for the time being let it remain a laboratory curiosity requiring further research.

Finding a lump

When we were young and sat around in a circle in the dark telling ghost stories, it did not take long before we were so primed and tightly-strung that any sudden noise or strange sound filled us with fear, and we would jump with fright at the smallest movement. This was a process of 'fright conditioning', where we expected the very worst and reacted accordingly.

In many ways finding a breast lump also triggers an automatic fright response. It is something women dread. Stories in the press and magazines, television documentaries about movie stars and young women in their prime — all sorts of dreadful accounts of the horrors of cancer leave women feeling sensitized and vulnerable.

Reactions

With this kind of background-conditioning scenario, finding a lump is likely to make you worried and frightened. It does not necessarily help much to hear that only one in ten lumps (or less) will turn out

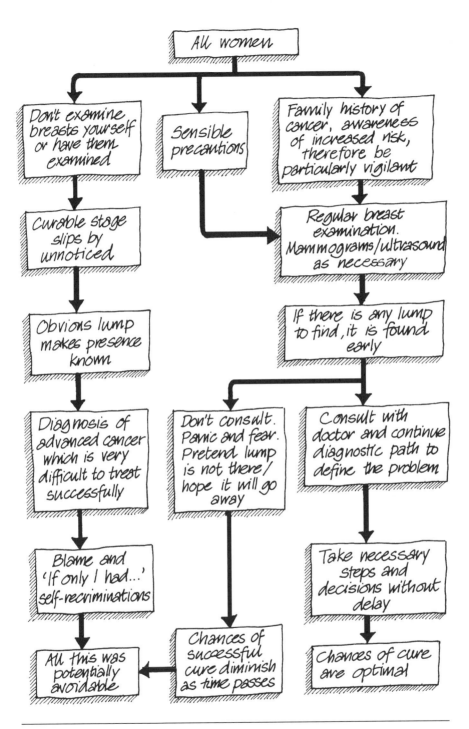

Figure 4.2 *Detecting a breast lump*

to be malignant. So with this overpowering, gut-wrenching fear, what can be done? Ignore it and it will go away? 'Yes that's it! It is not really there after all, so why worry?' The old concept of an ostrich with its head in the sand is understandable but it is very dangerous. The tragedy is that this attitude solves nothing, causes delay, reduces the options available, and may cost you your life.

I remember that as a child I knew for months that I had a cavity in a tooth. My tongue told me it was getting bigger, but my mind kept putting off taking the positive step of actually going to see the dentist. When, finally, there was no choice but to go, the tooth was in such bad shape that expensive and extensive repair work had to be done to save it. I had a relaxing feeling of relief having at last gone and done what I had put off for months. During those months I had never been completely at ease in any case, knowing what I needed to do.

The risk of delay is many times greater — and potentially life-threatening — as regards a lump. One tragedy is not looking for and not finding cancer if it is there; but perhaps worse is the tragedy of finding it and doing nothing about it until it may be too late.

Other symptoms that need urgent attention

Apart from the finding of a breast lump, there are other signs or symptoms that demand urgent medical attention. They are not always serious, but must be fully investigated:

- discharge (especially if bloody) from the nipple;
- dimpling or inward pulling down of the skin of the breast in a local area;
- lump (gland) in the armpit;
- changes in the skin of the breast, when it feels thicker and looks like the skin of an orange, with more obvious pores;
- ulceration of the breast skin (without having hurt it) that does not heal;
- persistent pain in the breast (rare form of painful cancer).

If you find a lump in your breast,
see a doctor straight away.

66 *Some delays are inherent in the medical system, with further assessment, tests, and biopsies. This makes it all the more important that you don't delay in seeking help if you find something in your breast that bothers you.* **John** **99**

Chapter 5

The steps to a diagnosis

Approach to finding a lump (see Figure 5.1)

The first and most important aspect is that looking for a breast lump must always be regarded as positive action. The fear of finding one must never be allowed to outweigh the conscious belief that the sooner it is found, the better the prospects will be for the future. While finding a lump in your breast is the last thing you *want* to happen, if it is there it must be detected as soon as possible. You cannot afford to ignore the fact that six or seven out of ten women will detect a lump in their breast at some time in their lives. In most cases, without a biopsy there can be no certainty about the character of the lump. One in ten women will develop breast cancer, and of these more than half will die within five years. However, in women whose cancers are found early and while still *in situ*, almost 100% will be alive five years later. The only sure way of improving your chances is early detection.

Most surveys reveal that only about 25% of women examine their own breasts or have them examined on a regular basis. This situation must be improved upon.

When or how are lumps found? (see Figure 5.2)

Between 70 and 80% of breast lumps are found by the woman herself. As screening mammography in asymptomatic patients grows in popularity and is more widely used, so the proportion of breast cancer detected in this fashion will increase. Self-palpation is still crucial to the process of detection, so it is difficult to understand anyone advocating mammograms replacing breast self-examination. The two methods should go hand-in-hand rather than one replacing the other.

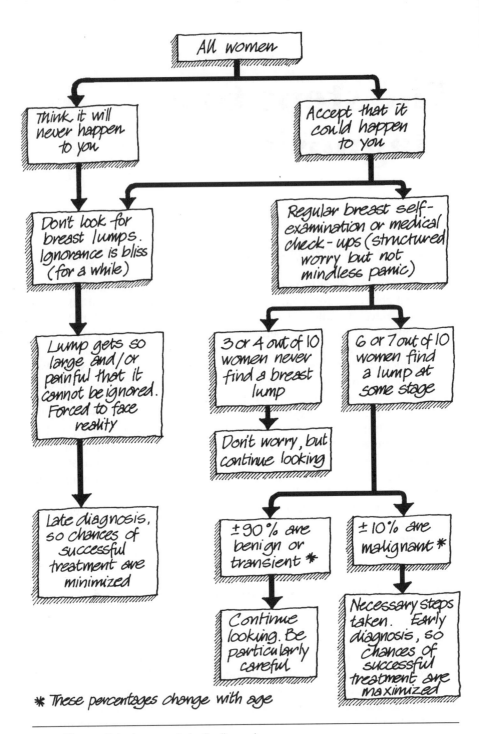

Figure 5.1 *Approach to finding a lump*

Once the lump is found (see Figure 5.2)

There is only one sensible path to follow after finding a lump, and that is to consult your doctor directly and then take whatever further steps are deemed necessary. Trying to ignore the lump and hoping (or praying) that it will go away may well lead to an avoidable tragedy. Sadly, many women present with advanced disease, and when questioned about the lump admit having known about it for weeks, months, or even years!

Consulting a doctor (see Figure 5.3)

First, a doctor will take a history from you, including your family history, pregancies, oral contraception, when the lump was noticed and whether it has changed since you found it. He will want to know the current stage of your menstrual cycle or pregnancy. He will examine you fully, and then depending on what he finds, the nature of your breast tissue, the nature of the lump, and the phase of your menstrual cycle, he will offer you various options. If the lump is an obvious one and has not changed through a menstrual cycle he may suggest a biopsy at once. More likely he will request a mammogram, or he may refer you to a surgical colleague for an opinion, in which case a second doctor will take your history again and do another examination. Probably you will still end up having a mammogram or an ultrasound scan (US).

Aspiration

If the lump is cystic (not solid), it may be aspirated by the ultrasonographer or radiologist under 'direct' vision (US or X-ray). This is an accurate and not-too-uncomfortable method. It may also be done by the surgeon who palpates (feels) the lump and then aspirates it. Usually this does not require even a local anaesthetic. If the cyst is seen to collapse down completely on US or X-ray, and if the fluid aspirated is clear, then that is all there is to it. If the fluid is bloody it will be sent for histology, to look for cancer cells, but even then cancer is very unlikely.

Biopsy

If the lump is solid, it requires a biopsy. I strongly advocate against the old-fashioned approach of 'watching it', even if the patient is under 40 years of age. If this is your doctor's opinion, I would suggest that at the very least you get a second opinion on the decision.

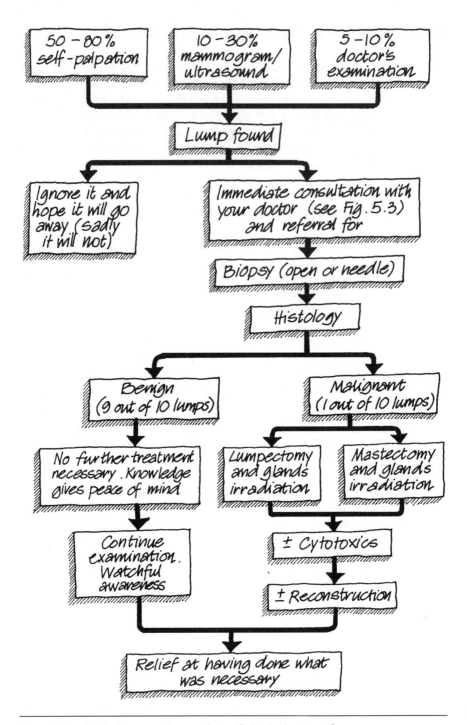

Figure 5.2 *How are lumps found? And what next?*

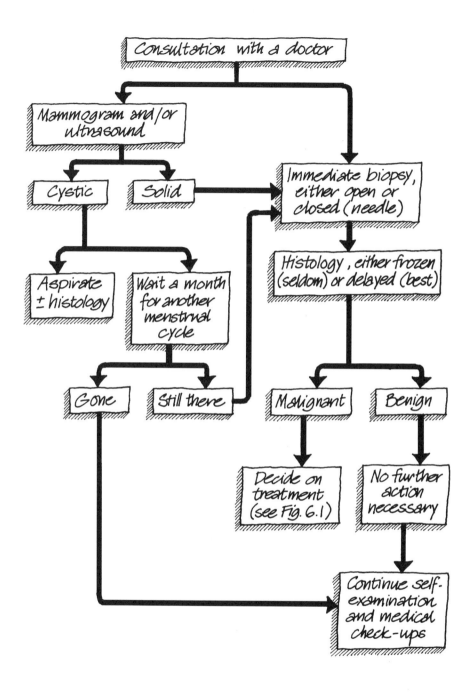

Figure 5.3 *Steps to take after finding a lump*

The only safe lump is a biopsied one. This biopsy may take two forms:

A needle biopsy can be done using a small aspiration (suction) needle or by means of a larger 'cutting' biopsy needle. The material obtained is sent for histology in both cases.

An open biopsy may take the form of a wedge (piece) biopsy if the lump is large, or it may be an excision biopsy (total removal or lumpectomy) if it is small. For an open biopsy a small surgical incision (cut) will be made and a drain (to allow blood and fluid to escape) may be left in after the lump has been excised. This stops blood and lymph accumulating in the space the lump was removed from and prevents a possible haematoma (blood clot) and infection occurring locally.

Most of these procedures are done in the surgeon's surgery, but it may be more convenient or necessary to use a hospital or clinic theatre.

What is a frozen section?

This technique was used to freeze tissue, cut it very thinly, and do the histology immediately, while the patient remained anaesthetized. The old horror stories of going into theatre for a biopsy, having a frozen section on the table and waking up mutilated (as if attacked by a shark) following a radical mastectomy are now part of the evolutionary history of breast-cancer management. As knowledge of the way cancer grows and spreads has increased, so the extent of mastectomy surgery has been modified and reduced. Now curative surgery is offered as a two-stage procedure — there is no dramatic urgency to carry out a frozen-section biopsy with immediate removal of the breast, as occurred in the past.

Stage one

- Biopsy and diagnosis are positive for cancer.
- Discussion and planning with doctor, family, and friends.
- Decision as to whether to have a lumpectomy or mastectomy, after going through the pros and cons of the procedures (see Table 6.1 on pages 62–3).
- Preparation for surgery (mental preparation and acceptance stage).

Stage two

- Booked and planned as a non-emergency but urgent surgical procedure, following on the preparation and discussion stage.
- Surgery will require hospital or clinic admission for either lumpectomy or mastectomy, with lymph node (glands) removal for staging purposes. Staging is a very important step, as this determines the nature and duration of futher treatment and management options.

After the biopsy — the waiting

There can be few situations in life which compare with the anxiety and worry evoked during this period of waiting. Fortunately with modern histological and staining techniques (to see the cell type and character), the result is usually available a day or two after the biopsy was taken. A restless, sleepless night while you lie awake imagining every conceivable negative prospect you can think of is the level of worry you may experience during this stage. While you try in vain to convince yourself that nine out of ten biopsied lumps turn out to be benign, there is always a little voice that says, 'Ah yes, but you are the exception, you are the one.' There are very few words of consolation or support that help during this stage, because very few people can imagine what you are trying to come to grips with. In fact you yourself don't even know yet, but you probably feel terrified.

Knowing about friends, relatives, or aquaintances who had negative (benign) results from biopsies does not seem to help; the mind conjures up vivid, gloomy images. You race way ahead of reality as your imagination leap-frogs over any common-sense barriers you try to place in its path. I don't know of any way to reduce the worry, except to repeat that nine out of ten women in these circumstances will be worrying needlessly.

The news — benign or malignant?

The surgeon will usually want to examine the biopsy site and/or remove the drain if it was an open biopsy, and so will usually see you at his rooms. At this time he will discuss the biopsy result with you. If you had a needle biopsy, he may inform you by telephone that it is benign or ask you to come and see him. You usually know whether the news is bad by his face and body language when you come into the consulting room. If he tells you the result is positive for cancer you will feel as if the bottom has fallen out of your world.

No matter how well-prepared you are for bad news, there will be a feeling of utter disbelief and incomprehension that such a disaster could possibly have happened to you. You will almost certainly cry, and will tend at this stage to take in very little more of what he may try to tell you.

Your mind will be in a turmoil, and I cannot emphasize it strongly enough that your husband, lover, a friend, or family member must accompany you to the doctor. The presence and support of someone you feel close to will be invaluable. He or she is more likely to take in what the doctor is saying or suggesting as a plan of action. Now is not the time for you to discuss in any detail the options open to you. You are in a state of shock and you may respond with passive disbelief or aggressive anger. You need to go home and gather your loved-ones around to protect and comfort you during this vulnerable period. The next chapter deals with the discussion stage and with the options available.

If the biopsy turned out to be negative (not cancer), you can return to your normal life somewhat shaken but happy, relieved, and determined to continue with your vigilant approach.

**The one thing worse than
finding breast cancer early
is finding it late.**

The face of fear

When, after the frightening wait, the diagnosis is finally made
And you are so apprehensive and very much afraid
And you want like a child to cry, scream, stamp, and agressively
  shout
And you lash out at those who love you and you throw your weight
  about
These reactions are normal and must not cause you additional pain
As denial, anger, fear, and frustration are part of the initial strain
But this kaleidoscope of reactions that seem to cause more strife
Help you regain equilibrium and then to plan for the rest of your life.

***Fear is a normal response
but to be controlled.***

      *On being told that I had breast cancer after my biopsy
proved positive, I experienced a feeling of utter disbelief
and despair. Any further meaningful planning of what
should or could be done was impossible until hours later.*
Jenny

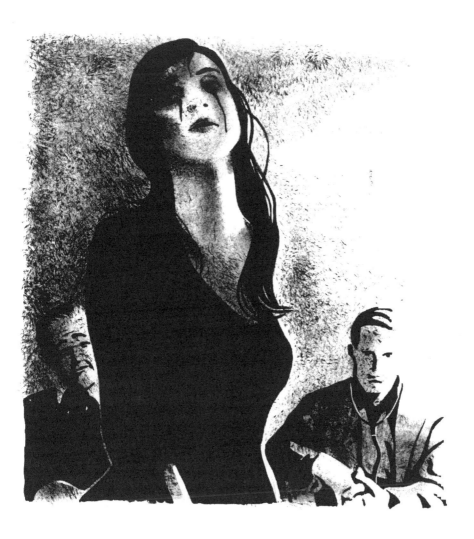

Chapter 6

After the diagnosis and before surgery

Thoughts about losses and gains

Whenever you are feeling down, repeat this to yourself.

> *Without life's downs I would not appreciate upward gain*
> *And well-being cannot be judged if I have known no pain*
> *Sadly, the precious aspects of living my everyday life*
> *Tended to be lost as I focused on small moments of strife*
> *But now, after waging the battle against cancer and fear,*
> *I can embrace life fully and with a heartfelt and glorious cheer*
> *See everything more clearly, and certainly in better perspective*
> *As I am rewarded with another chance, I must in turn be reflective.*

> **For every down I**
> **must create an up.**

Discussion with your doctor

Some preliminary discussion may have taken place when you were informed of the positive biopsy result. For some women who were in strong control of their emotions this may have been constructive. I feel that for most patients a two-phase discussion is necessary: short and brief on making the diagnosis, and then longer and more detailed once the patient has had time to assimilate the reality of both the diagnosis and its consequences.

Many doctors are very kind and understanding and have all the empathy required. Others may not seem to be as sympathetic. What must be remembered is that they can only judge through their own experience what may be worrying you and what specifically they think you should know; from your point of view, remember that you are an individual and that specific questions you do not ask may well remain unanswered. You have the right to be fully informed about your options (see Figure 6.1), so ask questions and find out all you want to know. There are pros and cons to both mastectomy and lumpectomy (see Table 6.1). The roles of cytotoxics, radiation therapy, and future reconstruction options are covered in more detail in Chapters 9 and 10. These aspects may be discussed by your doctor while various treatment options are under consideration.

Question time

For any patient who is seeing a doctor to discuss a complex issue such as the treatment for breast cancer, I suggest drawing up a list of questions beforehand. This is much like a shopping-list: we have all experienced the frustration of going shopping without a complete list but with certain items in mind, only to return home without the things we wanted. In exactly the same way, write down all the questions which for you are worrying, unclear, or incompletely explained and then go through them in detail, step-by-step, with your doctor (like a shopping list) until you are completely satisfied.

What is best for me?

There are many aspects to consider when deciding on what form of treatment is best for you. They include your age, the size of your breasts, the size and type of the tumour, its exact whereabouts, and signs of spread. None of these factors is decisive in isolation. In addition, the advice and belief of your surgeon as to what in his experience is the best option for you under the prevailing conditions is important, and his suggestions should be taken into account. If after

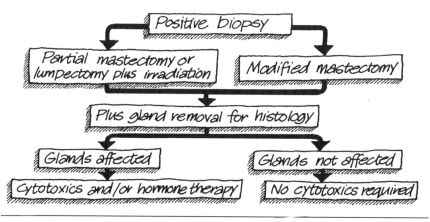

Figure 6.1 *Mastectomy options*

discussing the options you are still unsure, and would like a second opinion, then it is your right to ask for one. Most doctors are perfectly happy with this, as the ultimate aim is to have a patient who is confident of having chosen the right form of treatment.

I cannot tell you what is considered the best form of management, in view of the many variables involved. What I will say is that in my wife's case we chose a modified mastectomy, as she was young (40) and I was not sure about long-term risks of radiation therapy. In addition, in her case a second and third ductal carcinoma was present in other quadrants of the breast, which would have been left behind if we had chosen a lumpectomy. Note that I have spoken of 'we' and not 'she', as this was a joint decision. How significant the other *in situ* carcinomas would have turned out to be — whether they would ever have become invasive — we will never know. With lumpectomy, radiation is mainly directed at the tumour bed (the area it was removed from), and whether it would have eradicated the other cancers is something we will never know.

On the other hand, follow-up studies are showing that for the same stage of disease, lumpectomy with gland removal followed by cytotoxics (if necessary) and radiation is resulting in outcomes as good as (and in some instances better than) mastectomy. There is no easy answer. The advice of an experienced surgeon should be sought, and given full consideration before you decide to opt for an alternative form of surgery. The surgeon with the most detailed knowledge of your case does generally know what is best for you. For younger women who may wish to breast-feed children, this should also be taken into consideration when the various options are considered. The only irrefutable fact is that you must have surgical removal of the cancer — remember the comparison with towing away most of the hot-rod cancer cars and then destroying the rest with cytotoxics and/or radiation. Only very elderly women and women with very advanced cancer should consider receiving hormone and cytotoxic therapy without the benefit of surgery.

What types of surgery are performed?

Excision biopsy (mini-lumpectomy)

In this case the small lump is totally removed (as determined on histology) at the time of doing an open diagnostic biopsy. It should still be followed by gland removal to determine that they are clear of spread, and then radiation treatment should be given to the biopsy area. This form of excision biopsy with total removal is uncommon because most diagnosis is now done using a needle biopsy.

Lumpectomy (with gland removal) and radiation

It is generally agreed that lumpectomy alone without gland removal is a very risky approach. Lumpectomy involves surgical removal of the lump with some surrounding breast tissue (this usually spares the nipple, but not always) as well as removing the glands from the axilla. It is always followed by radiation therapy. If the glands are clear (on histology), radiation therapy commences two weeks after surgery (to allow scar healing) and continues for six weeks. If the glands are not clear, then cytotoxics are given first and followed by radiation after about six weeks of cytotoxic treatment.

Partial mastectomy (with gland removal)

Here part of the breast (the quadrant containing the cancer) is removed, or almost all of the breast tissue but with preservation of skin and nipple. Glands are again removed, sometimes through a separate incision. Reconstruction is easier, but leaving behind some breast tissue and the nipple may increase future risks. There is also an increased risk of skin or nipple necrosis (tissue death) due to lack of blood supply following the operation where skin and nipple are retained but breast tissue is removed.

Modified mastectomy (with gland removal)

In this instance the whole breast — skin, nipple, and axillary (armpit) glands — is removed. What must be stressed is that *it is not a radical mastectomy*, which involved removing the large muscles of the chest wall and which left a disfiguring scar much like a shark-attack victim. This is 'merely' breast and gland-tissue removal, and leaves the chest muscles intact and available for having a silicone bag implanted behind them for reconstruction purposes. Arm strength is preserved, and most sports can still be played.

Only with the lumpectomy forms of surgery is further radiation therapy indicated, as total clearance of all the cancer cannot be guaranteed. In all forms of surgery any further treatment with cytotoxics is directly determined by whether or not the axillary glands are involved.

Putting memory ghosts to rest

Images from days gone by, of women who had undergone radical mastectomies, linger on and contribute to the horrendous picture of breast-cancer surgery that many women conjure up. Such radical

Lumpectomy (plus gland removal)	Glands involved so cytotoxics required. This delays irradiation by 6 weeks
	Irradiation
	Less disfiguring
	Less post-operative pain and discomfort
	Shorter post-operative recovery period
	Possibility that original cancer removal incomplete, requiring further surgery (see below)
	May have left a second cancer behind
	5 –10% will still require a mastectomy in next 5 years due to recurrence.
	Reconstruction easier and more aesthetically pleasing
	Five-year survival same as mastectomy (may even be better)
	Irradiation in younger women may increase long-term cancer risk in exposed breast and lung tissue
	Irradiation may be frightening for some people and may cause local breast or chest pain (rib fracture) or radiation inflammation of lungs
	Irradiation as an ongoing process for 2 months extends the 'reminder period' — continue going to cancer radiation clinic
	More acceptable concept to most women, especially in the 20–40 age group
	The 'in vogue' operation and therefore women are likely to be happy with it
	Arm swelling (lymph drainage decreased due to gland resection and radiation therapy)

Table 6.1 *The pros and cons of lumpectomy and modified mastectomy*

Modified mastectomy (plus gland removal)	Glands involved so cytotoxics required.
	No irradiation
	More disfiguring
	More post-operative pain and discomfort
	Longer post-operative recovery period
	All primary cancer and breast tissue removed (as far as possible)
	All cancer sites in that breast removed
	Mastectomy already done
	Reconstruction may be more difficult and less aesthetically pleasing (good results are possible)
	Five-year survival same as lumpectomy
	No irradiation, so no increased long-term potential risk for younger women
	No further frightening experience and no further discomfort once healed
	No ongoing 'reminder period' — need not attend cancer radiation clinics
	Less acceptable concept to most women
	Has been the gold standard in the past but now is often matched by lumpectomy and therefore may seem unnecessary
	Arm swelling (lymph drainage reduced due to gland resection)

surgery is hardly ever indicated nowadays and these lingering memories must be erased. They are very far from the reality of modern surgery followed by effective cosmetic reconstruction.

Decisions about breast cancer start by being difficult and don't become any easier.

What are the costs involved?

The first 'cost' you will pay is losing your peace of mind. After having breast cancer diagnosed, your life changes forever: you will always worry about new symptoms or signs; 'normal' aches and pains become instant causes for alarm. This degree of worry diminishes as the number of false alarms increases, but it never goes away completely. It is indeed a high price to pay.

Finances

While this may seem an odd aspect to be considering at this early stage of the proceedings, it is one of many factors that need to be taken into consideration.

Depending on your financial status, medical aid cover, and insurance, many courses of action are open to you. These also depend on the health-care system of your country, on what facilities are provided by the state, and what private facilities are available.

Some general points:
- Medical aid societies differ as to what they cover and the extent of cover provided. For example, some may consider breast reconstruction as cosmetic surgery and therefore not cover such costs. Find out before embarking on a course of action what costs are covered, to what degree, and of course what is not covered at all. This avoids nasty surprises when the final accounts are submitted for payment.
- For those who have an insurance policy which covers breast cancer, remember to check the small print carefully. Most such policies cover only the initial diagnosis and treatment, and do do not cover subsequent developments such as secondary spread with accompanying complications and further treatment.
- Travel insurance does not cover problems arising as a result of breast cancer diagnosed prior to travelling, be it days, weeks, months, or years before.
- Costs of private medical care are high, especially in private hospitals. If you are not on medical aid and will be financially

strained or embarrassed by such costs, remember that state hospitals — certainly in the bigger centres — usually provide excellent care and management. Facilities may be more crowded than in private hospitals, and not always as comfortable, but quality of surgery and treatment is usually top-class.

■ The same applies should you require further chemotherapy (cytotoxics). Such care should ideally be planned and managed by a radiation oncologist attached to the breast-cancer clinic of a state hospital. Such personnel usually have the knowledge and experience to determine what therapy is best for you in your particular situation. In certain centres this may be available through large private hospitals.

So while your health remains the most important factor and cannot ever be compared to 'mere money', there are various options open to you. These should be considered carefully. To be financially crippled through the devastating condition of breast cancer is an additional strain at a time when stress needs to be minimized. There is more than enough to cope with without being burdened by unnecessary financial crises.

    66 *I have never regretted having to lose my breast, as that meant gaining my life. What I have regretted is that I was unfortunate enough to have had breast cancer, and what it has done to my peace of mind.* **Jenny** **99**

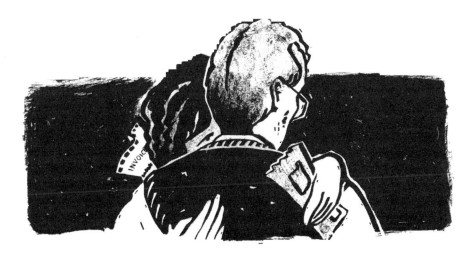

Chapter 7

Preparing for hospitalization and surgery

Getting ready for hospitalization

It is often easier in life to face the known than the unknown. By this stage you have accepted the fact that you have breast cancer and that some form of surgery is inevitable. (The only other option is to refuse surgery and rely on natural remedies and prayer. I don't consider this a viable alternative pathway. Prayer can always help you along the path of surgical and other medical treatment, and faith can be a wonderful support throughout treatment and convalescence. I don't think that faith and medicine should ever be mutually exclusive.)

With your doctor's guidance you have decided on what form the surgery will take, so now is the time for strengthening your mental resolve. The power of positive thinking must be firmly established by the time you go to hospital. Do not bottle up fears and misgivings — discuss them with a loved-one, a friend, or even contact someone who has been through the ordeal you are facing. Keep on asking any questions that worry you, even though they may seem trivial.

When you know something unpleasant is unavoidable there is still a tendency to put it last in the pecking-order of all the other things that suddenly seem so important to do right now. While immediate surgery is not an absolute emergency, it must be done soon. Some collective thought and preparation time is acceptable, but do not procrastinate too long — it does not become any easier.

If you are leaving a home where your partner, children, or domestic help can continue with the normal routine of running the household, then not much organization by you will be necessary. If, on the other hand, everything will come to an abrupt halt when you go into hospital, quite a lot of planning and preparation will have to

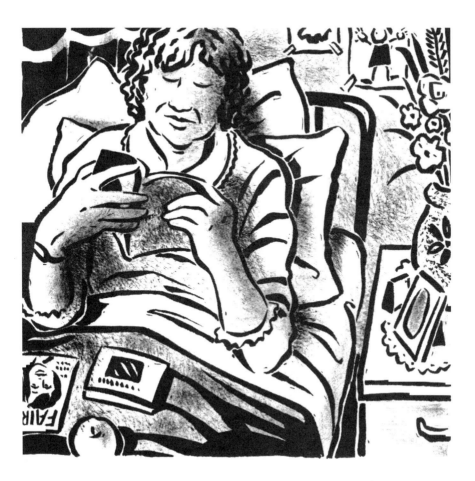

be done. If you live either alone or with only your children, then remember to attend to the following:

- Organize for your children to stay with friends or relatives.
- Cancel milk and papers.
- Alert neighbours and police. Perhaps leave a light on.
- Organize for someone to feed any pets and water plants.
- Leave your key with a friend or relative so that they have access in an emergency, or to fetch anything you find you need.
- Stock up on non-perishable groceries for your return (friends then need only buy you perishable goods).
- Contact a home-nursing service (if you can afford one), or make arrangements for a friend or relative to come and stay with you when you return. Knowing they will be there for you will give you peace of mind.
- Arrange who will take you to hospital and who will fetch you.

What to tell children

Depending on the age of your children, you should tell them as much of the truth as they can understand. For the very young (three to five-year-olds), probably say only that you are going to hospital for an operation. For the somewhat older child (say, six to nine), tell them that you will be having a breast operation; and for those with more understanding (say, ten upwards), mention that it is for breast cancer. Once again, honesty and openness is the best approach. Hidden things become secretive things, and thus more frightening than if they are discussed openly.

Strengthening relationships

This is a crucial time for developing the understanding and support-ive relationship between your partner (husband/lover) and yourself. Remember that to him, too, this diagnosis is an enormous shock, and that he needs to adapt to the concept. He loves you and wants to help. These efforts to help may be constructive or extremely clumsy. He may feel so awkward or be so unsure of his role that he will seem to be 'withdrawn'.

This cocoon of silence and withdrawal must not be allowed to develop. Despite all the responsibility and worry that you are already carrying, you may have to take the lead in encouraging him to talk about what is worrying him. It is no good saying to yourself, 'Look what I am having to face! Can't he even support me like a man?' This hostile attitude will set you on paths destined to take you further apart rather than bring you closer together.

On the other hand, your partner may be mature enough and confident enough in his male role to express his love, caring, and concern for you, and he may discuss the problem quite openly.

He will be able to put the possible loss of a breast in perspective and to express his total love for you-the-person rather than for you-with-nice-breasts. These supportive approaches may be open and strong or exploratory and tentative. Whichever is the case, they must be accepted, and encouraged to take firm root, and be culti-vated. This support is then sure to bear fruit in the trying time ahead.

Not every woman will have a husband or lover currently in her life, but there will always be family or special friends. The renewing or strengthening of relationships with such loved-ones becomes even more important when you have breast cancer. Their support and understanding acts as a buffer: they don't stop the knocks, but they soften the blows. Their protective value is enormous in helping you adjust to the prospect of surgery.

You, too, have an important role to play in developing these supportive relationships. Each person is governed by his or her own personality, degree of shyness, and concepts of femininity. This will effect the 'openness' of any discussions and determine how far you can comfortably go. The moral here is: 'Go as far as you possibly can along the path of honesty and frankness and then a little further!' Push yourself. So often when something is finally out in the open it becomes much easier to speak about it. Eventually you may even laugh about your own particular hang-ups.

So this phase before surgery is one for strengthening morale and relationships. You are laying the foundation on which you will build further coping strategies as you face other hurdles such as reconstruction or further treatment with cytotoxics or radiation. It is a very important stage, and not merely an in-limbo-with-fear gap between diagnosis and surgery.

What to expect in hospital

Few people can enter a hospital without a degree of apprehension or even dislike. Hospitals conjure up memories — real or imagined — which have been etched into our subconscious through actual experiences, films, books, and magazine articles.

The décor in modern hospitals and clinics tends to be much better than in older ones. Newer buildings often have flowers, pictures or murals, and walls painted in more pleasing and relaxing colours. You may, however, be having your surgery done in an older-style hospital rather than a modern clinic. Please remember that it is the doctors, nurses, and paramedical staff who are important rather than the décor — the quality of a present is not determined by the wrapping paper!

If possible, arrange to be admitted early on the morning of your surgery rather than the night before; depending on the hospital and the anaesthetist this is often possible. Any blood tests required before anaesthesia can be done on an outpatient basis. This saves you the ordeal of lying awake, frightened, facing surgery the next day, in an environment that is not as familiar and comforting as your own home. If this is not possible, then do your best to accept what cannot be changed.

Let the 'h' in hospital stand for
hope, help, health, and happiness.

What to take to hospital

This will vary depending on what is important to you as a person. You may want to look especially feminine and attractive, in which case make-up, hair accessories, and attractive bed-jackets and pyjamas are the order of the day. On the other hand, such things may not be important to you. Take photographs of loved-ones, family, and friends, as these can be very comforting. If you have a particular good-luck charm or something that reminds you of a particularly happy or memorable occasion, certainly take that too. Take your book of worship if you use one.

Other things that may help with recovery:

- Take your favourite tapes and a walkman — borrow one if need be.
- Buy yourself that book you have always wanted to read but never found the time to, or at least buy a selection of your favourite magazines.
- Take with you, or ask family and friends to bring you, your favourite specialities to eat. Spoil yourself!
- Continue your 'shopping list' of questions. There are bound to be new ones you want to ask medical staff, so take pen and paper to jot them down as they occur to you.

The hospital routine

Make a friend of the ward sister. Introduce yourself to her and familiarize yourself with the ward routine. There will be many occasions when she can help answer your queries and may also be able to allay your fears. Do the same with night staff and get to know them as individuals who can help and support you. Simple things such as knowing about meal-times, visiting times, whether you can receive telephone calls, waking-up times, and availability of toilet and bathroom facilities will all help to reassure you.

Routine observations and tests will continue. These may include blood tests, urine tests, and taking your temperature and pulse regularly. Blood tests are routine before an anaesthetic, so don't worry about them — they may even have been done the day before you were admitted.

Going to theatre

You will be given nil per mouth (NPM) for at least six hours before surgery. In preparation for going to theatre you will be asked to put on a rather unflattering theatre gown instead of your own pyjamas or dressing-gown. All jewellery will have to be removed, including rings, as you cannot wear any tight objects while under anaesthesia. This may be upsetting, especially having to take off rings with a strong emotional significance, such as a wedding ring. All nail polish and lipstick will have to be removed so that the anaesthetist can see the true colour of your nail-beds and lips. In addition, a floppy, shapeless cap may be put over your hair. You may not look your most attractive on your way to theatre, but don't let that worry you. If the situation were not so fraught with anxiety, and if you could view it from a distance, it would even have its humourous side! You will normally have been given a 'pre-med' — a form of sedation with an agent to dry up body secretions — so your mouth (which may already have been dry due to apprehension) will feel even drier. Your armpit will also have been shaved on the side you are having surgery.

So off you go, trying your best to hold back the tears, but not always succeeding. Your husband or a loved-one or close friend should be there to hold your hand as they wheel you to theatre on a trolley. Letting go of that supportive hand, and the last glimpse of the anxious face of the person who loves you and has come to support you will be tough, and the tears may well start to roll then. Don't worry about it — crying is a perfectly natural and acceptable reaction.

Once in theatre, the lights and instrumentation, staff and anaesthetist will only be seen for a short while before you drift off under the effect of the anaesthetic agent, usually administered directly into a vein. This 'puts you to sleep' quickly, and then anaesthesia is maintained with anaesthetic gases administered through a tube into your upper airway (trachea). You may therefore wake up with a slightly hoarse voice and sore throat as a result of the tube.

After the operation

Well, it's all over. Not quite in fact, but it often feels that way. There is a sense of relief at the removal of a millstone that you have been carting around. You will be sleepy and and a little confused from the anaesthetic. It is essential that when you get back to the ward your husband, family, or a close friend is there to welcome you. At this stage you will probably give them a brave smile, squeeze a hand or two, and then drift off into a well-deserved sleep.

What about pain?

Yes, the days after your operation will be painful and uncomfortable, but at no stage unbearable. What is most important for you to understand is that you need not endure any excessive pain. You know it is going to be sore, so as the effects of the anaesthetic wear off, and before it gets very painful, do something to get the pain under control. The more pain and discomfort you allow to develop, the more tense and unhappy you will become. Pain can be blocked, so use the modern drugs available. Ask for them early, if they have not already been given to you. Do not try to be brave and to grin and bear it — it proves nothing, solves nothing, and creates unecessary additional problems. Unfortunately some doctors and nursing staff may not be fully aware of the need to prevent pain reaching a certain threshold, so even if you have been prescribed pain-killers (analgesics), they may only be given when you complain of severe pain. I want you to request them *before* you have severe pain. The discomfort can and must be minimized. You have enough adjusting to do without having to endure pain unnecessarily.

So what now? — Mindpower

You *must* be determined to put on a good show. You must approach recovery in a positive and 'I-know-I-can-jolly-well-do-it' frame of mind. Do not allow yourself to withdraw into a shell of self-pity — tempting though this may be. This is the first stage of the rest of your life: set the trend and make it positive. There will be times when in the quiet of your hospital room you will want to hug a loved-one, cling to him or her, and silently weep. That's fine; but then you must dry the tears, grit your teeth, and say, 'I can and will overcome this!' Do not try to do it alone. Open up to your husband, lover, family members or friends, depending on your particular circumstances. Let them in, let them share, let them support, and it will help to sooth your emotional wound and to heal it more quickly.

Other points not to worry about

■ You may still have an intravenous drip for a while. This is normal, and only slightly uncomfortable — more of a nuisance really, as it limits your arm movements.

- You may have rubber or plastic tubes draining the chest wound. These may increase the discomfort and awkwardness of moving.
- There may be numbness behind your shoulder and down into your arm, depending on the cutaneous (skin) nerves that were cut during gland removal. This improves with time.
- There may be a tingling and burning sensation of the chest due to the small cutaneous nerves that were cut. This also improves with time.
- With movement, the wound and stitches will pull and be sore, but because the chest muscles have not been cut, the pain of movement is not as severe as you expect it to be — one bonus point!
- Routine post-op observations will be done on you. This is not because medical staff are particularly worried about you, or because anything is necessarily wrong, but simply to ensure that no unexpected problems arise.
- Even though it *feels* as though the wound is pulling apart when you move, this will not happen, so do not be afraid to move gently.

Convalescing

The meaning of the word 'convalesce' is 'the gradual recovery of health and strength' and is derived from the Latin — meaning 'to be strong'. In this case, strength refers to strength of mind, strength of soul, and strength of resolve and character. Although strictly speaking you can only convalesce once you have had your surgery, I feel that the process of recovery starts before surgery. This is linked to your outlook, determination, and power of positive thinking. If before surgery you have been able to accept what is unavoidable, and adapt to what is going to happen to you, then with the love and support of family and friends the recovery phase will be easier and shorter, and can even be viewed as a new challenge in your life. Certainly, it is a challenge you would rather have done without, but there are events in our lives which we have little or no control over. So start getting better in your mind *before* surgery. Work at it!

When will you go home?

This depends a lot on you, your home circumstances, your support group, your type of surgery, and your doctor's attitude to early or later discharge. For some, going home quickly is very important and is something they strive for. For others, staying in hospital a while longer to be cared and catered for until they are feeling considerably better is a more acceptable approach. Different patients will recover more slowly or quickly than others who have undergone the same surgery. Attitude, strength of mind, and pain thresholds (all of which can vary widely from one individual to another) affect this process. By the time you go home, drains have usually been removed but sutures (stitches) are still in.

On the day you leave hospital you will be saying goodbye to all the nursing and paramedical staff, and to other patients who you have grown fond of during your hospital stay. You are now well and truly taking the first important steps on the road to recovery and regaining your independence. In the hospital you were still in a protected environment — which is as it should be during your most painful, emotional, and vulnerable period. Now you are facing new challenges, and your strength of purpose must not waver.

Physiotherapy

This is of much greater importance for women who have undergone mastectomy than for those who have had a lumpectomy. The role of physiotherapy is fully described in Chapter 8, with suggestions about certain exercises to be done to keep the arm, and especially the shoulder joint, fully mobile.

Early physiotherapy and arm movement should be commenced in the hospital. Ideally a physiotherapist should see you, start you moving the 'sore' arm, and give you instructions regarding gentle exercises to begin with and others to graduate to later.

The physiotherapist often has a thankless task in life: no matter how kind, friendly, or pleasant the physiotherapist is, she has to make you do something uncomfortable and painful. If you do achieve the target she sets you, she will immediately set a new goal to be reached. This does not stop until you are back to normal — only then are you let off the hook!

Even though it is painful, try hard to move the arm and shoulder. It will seem much easier just to tuck the arm into your side and not move it, but this can have very serious consequences, with a 'frozen' shoulder joint and limitation of movement — a heavy price to pay for avoiding some discomfort early on. So this is another challenge that you must face in order to regain your full strength and arm mobility.

66 *By working at being a fine example you will help yourself recover. You will also gain the support of the nursing staff, which will help to make your hospital stay an easier one, and your positive attitude will make your family and friends feel happier. In addition you will help other women to be less frightened about having to face breast cancer.*
Jenny **99**

Chapter 8

The road to recovery

Returning home

You will only have been in hospital for a relatively short time — between two days and a week — but it may have felt longer if you have been longing to return home. It is at home that your next phase of recovery will take place, in surroundings that must be made as conducive to this as possible. Friends and family must be there to welcome you back with happy smiling faces — not serious, worried ones. Walking through your own front door will give you a feeling of having reached a rest-station after a long and tiring journey.

You may well be most comfortable in your own bed, but I would encourage you not to stay there too long. Being at rest does not necessarily mean being in bed. Arrange a comfortable reclining chair (borrow one if necessary), or use a comfortable couch in a room with a view. This should overlook the garden if you have one, but if not, choose the happiest room in the house, with as much light, flowers or plants, and sunshine as possible. Get properly dressed — do not stay in your night-clothes.

You will still be feeling very sore and sorry for yourself. During this recovery phase take pain-killers (analgesics) as necessary. Try to be within reach of a telephone. Do not isolate yourself: chat to friends; don't be shy or self-conscious; and try not to bottle up fears or misgivings. Your family and friends want to help and be involved, and are often waiting for signals from you. (It is also possible that they all become a nuisance and overtax you. You must not allow this to happen, so be firm when you want to rest: put the phone off the hook and a note on the front door saying 'Do not disturb now. Open for calls 4 pm. Looking forward to seeing you', or something in a similar vein.)

While you are recovering you will tire easily, and even simple things can feel like a big effort. Remember that if you cannot make

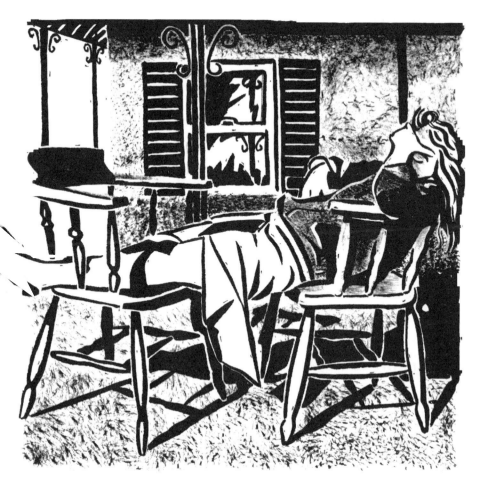

headway it is perfectly acceptable just to hold on for a while; but then try again — do not ever allow yourself to regress and go backwards. Remember that it is not only the happy things which pass in life; the unhappy things do too — and just as quickly. The essence of courage during this period is that even though your heart may quake sometimes, do not let other people be too aware of it. This takes great fortitude on your part, but in time will help you to feel emotionally and mentally stronger.

If your family or friends can rally and run the show for a while, excellent! The stress is on 'for a while', however. As soon as possible you should resume your former role and get involved in the running of your home. This will give you a feeling of accomplishment and is reassuring.

Home can be a haven to regain your health.

Recuperation

This is the stage of further healing and strengthening of physical form and mental resolve. Stitches come out after eight to ten days, and then moving about is a lot more comfortable. Physio and arm exercises are crucial during this stage (see later in this chapter). These must be established as a daily routine now and definitely not left until later 'when it won't be so sore'.

You may already have had an immediate reconstruction done at the time of the mastectomy, or you may be allowing time to heal first before deciding on a future course of action as regards a prosthesis or reconstruction.

Enjoy pets, family, and friends. In particular, try to revive or develop your sense of humour. Laughing and making light of things can be a very important part of the healing process and is also an important ingredient in most mature and worthwhile relationships. It is said that 'when there is a twinkle in the eye there is a spark of heaven in the heart'. (The role of humour and being able to see the lighter side of serious things is covered more fully in Chapter 11.)

Returning to work

Depending on home circumstances, financial needs, and security of employment, you may have to return to your job as soon as possible. Following a lumpectomy this should be possible two to three weeks after the operation, and with a modified mastectomy after four to six weeks.

Facing colleagues may be something you are secretly dreading — those knowing looks, whispered comments, and suddenly-halted conversation as you walk in all emphasize that you are the focus of their attention and discussion. How you handle it will depend a lot on your personality, but it is not an easy time. The more secretive you try to be, the more determined your colleagues will probably be to find out all the smallest details. So openness and honesty is still the best approach. Tell some of them what happened, give short explanatory answers to questions, and get back to your normal routine as soon as possible. The office grapevine will quickly disperse the information, and you will soon stop being the focus of inquisitive attention if you can adopt a matter-of-fact approach.

In a small, more personal office, where your colleagues are also your friends, much of the ice will have been broken by their visiting you in hospital or at home, so returning to such a work situation is much easier than to a big office.

Remember that while you do not ever have to reveal any intimate details or fears if you do not want to, talking frankly about your experience often puts an instant stop to inquisitive speculation. Be receptive to offers of help and support, which come in many guises — some awkward and tentative, others open and at times over-protective. Even if you feel they are unnecessary, see them for what they are — indications of concern for you — and accept such actions graciously. Many women may have their own covert fears of breast cancer, and the way you handle the situation can be both reassuring and a lesson to them.

Adjusting and acquiring confidence

Personalities are like kaleidoscopes: they have many of the same basic components, but the dominance of one component over another and what is seen when you look from different angles and at different times can vary tremendously. You may have adjusted well; you may have no need to regain your confidence, and you may have fully accepted what has happened to you. But for many women this does not come easily.

Confidence comes from within ourselves. It is based on past experience and on knowing what we can and cannot cope with. For some women, the disfiguring aspect of breast surgery, with potential loss of femininity and sexuality, may prove to be the biggest hurdle. For others, living with the threat of a cancer which may or may not have been completely cured is a constant sobering and limiting influence. For some, the question of their own mortality — living with the realization that there are no guarantees in life, and that tomorrow may not always be there for them — shakes them to the core of their being: dying is generally something we envisage happening much later on in our lives. Putting on a brave face can be such an effort that it leaves little energy for anything else. But many women, though frightened and shaken by the experience, grasp enthusiastically their good fortune at being given a second chance and get on with the business of living.

Convince yourself that you *can* be cured. Have full confidence in yourself and decide that you *can* cope. Coping is a must, but it is not an all-or-nothing situation: you are likely to be on an emotional see-saw, and the goal while having these ups and downs is to hang on. If you 'fall off' and give in to feeling low and depressed for long periods you will make the situation a lot worse.

Ongoing rehabilitation — mental attitude

The role of family and friends is extremely important during this phase, and is dealt with more fully in Chapter 11.

In many ways this period of recovery centres around you getting into perspective the sacrifices you have had to make and what you have gained by making them. Needless to say, such sacrifices were not optional. The first constructive lesson is that where there is no choice we do well to minimize the difficulty. This may sound glib, but if the alternative is considered — certain death — then the sacrifice of losing a breast or part of one, even taking into account the pain, suffering (emotional and physical), and any body image change, all pale in comparison. There is not really a comparison; the alternative is too final to contemplate.

The next point is strength of purpose. This starts in a small way, takes root, and thereafter can support you as it continues to grow. Do not try to develop the strength to see you through everything at once; treat it as a step-by-step process with goals you can achieve one by one.

Seemingly simple goals may in fact be quite difficult. The first one must be to get out of bed each morning, dress, do your hair, and apply whatever make-up you usually wear. Do not stay in bed feeling sorry for yourself. If you get tired, rest on a couch or in an easy chair — do not go back to bed. The next goal is to return to your normal daily routine as far as possible. Plan for your return to work, do things with your children, go shopping with a friend for your groceries (the friend can help with the physical work of carrying bags), and so on. Get back into the kitchen and cook, if that is what you usually do. Go out for short walks and gradually increase their length. Go out to see a show or a movie — do not just watch television or videos at home. Accept invitations from friends, rather than turning them down because you are scared of what people might say.

There will also be quiet moments for you to reflect and gain inner strength. Use these times to motivate yourself and to establish your priorities. Encourage yourself to put on a brave face even if you are still quaking inside.

Once you go out and meet people again, the awkwardness will start to recede. From here on you can continue to achieve new goals you set for yourself, such as learning a new language, doing a course at university or college, or taking up a new hobby such as cycling, pottery, dressmaking, yoga, or woodwork. The only limitation to what you can achieve is the mental barrier you erect — with effort and motivation you can surprise even yourself.

The most important message really is that minds govern bodies and not the other way round. Though you may worry at times about whether your cancer will recur in the future, try to be positive — it won't necessarily, and to spend your time worrying about it will spoil your life and affect those around you. A wise person who had experienced life and its problems in many guises once said, 'I have had many troubles in my life and most of them somehow never happened'.

Physiotherapy

Many trials have shown that both early physiotherapy and ongoing exercises are crucial ingredients for a full and speedy recovery. As most patients are only in hospital for about five days, it is important that physiotherapy is started immediately. Wound dehiscence (opening up) has not been a problem when a supervised early exercise schedule of arm and shoulder movement has been started. Earlier recovery and full return of shoulder movement was significantly better in mastectomy patients who had early, planned physiotherapy than it was in patients for whom physiotherapy was delayed until it was less uncomfortable.

Physiotherapy is not merely aimed at improving strength and movement. It is used specifically to achieve the following goals:
■ normal posture;
■ a full range of arm and shoulder movement;
■ regaining strength; and
■ lessening the degree of lymphoedema (swelling of the arm due to decreased lymphatic drainage).

The benefit of these aspects, as well as general physical well-being, also helps to improve mental attitude and determination. It provides an immediate goal which must be achieved, even though at times it may be extremely uncomfortable and will require perseverance and strength of character.

Posture
The natural tendency is to shield the area of pain and to bend over towards the side that was operated on. This often results in drooping of the shoulder on the affected side and bending of the spine. Such posture is termed 'protective splinting' — just as you splint a broken bone to stop it moving, so here you are 'splinting' an area that is painful to move and stretch. Tucking in the chin with shoulder elevation exercises, correction of posture while sitting, as well as

1   'Walking' up the wall using your fingers:
    a straight up in front of you while facing the wall;
    b out and up sideways, also while facing the wall.
    'Walk' as high as you can, and when painful 'walk' a tiny bit further. Mark this spot. The next time you do this you should reach the same spot, and try to get a little above or beyond it. Then mark a new spot.

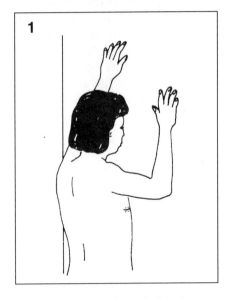

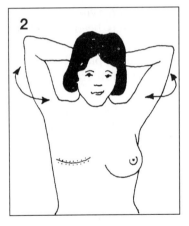

2   Put your hands up behind your head and try to clasp your hands. Once you can, swing your elbows gently forwards and backwards as if flying — get that broken wing working! Start slowly and increase the distance and force of the swing gradually.

3   Reach over your shoulder towards the small of your back from the top. Then reverse and try it again from the bottom. It will hurt, but keep trying — unless there is some discomfort you are not achieving anything. Dropping and catching a bean bag over your shoulder and behind your back is also a useful variation.

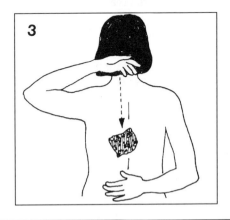

Figure 8.1 *Physiotherapy exercises once drains are removed*

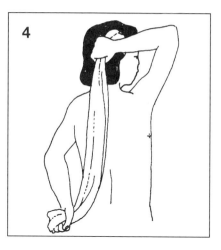

4   Use a towel (small) and dry your back. First one way, and then reverse top and bottom hands. (Instead of a towel, a wide piece of elastic or rubber can be gently stretched between your two hands.)

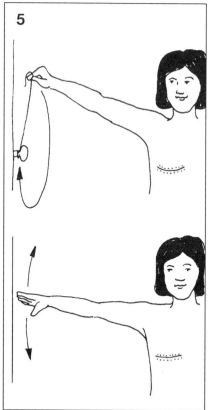

5   Full arm rotation: swing arm gently in small circles. It may help to tie a piece of string to a doorknob and swing around the knob in circles holding onto the string. Start with arm out sideways making small circles, and gradually move upwards until arm is vertical.

6   Depending on the weather and what pool or beach facilities are available, it often helps to get into water (once the stitches are out) and to use the resistance of the water to move your arm and shoulder against.

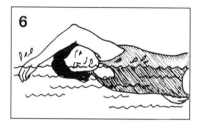

arm-swinging and good posture when walking are all helpful remedies. Heavy weights should not be carried on that side for about six to eight weeks.

Full range of motion

This is more difficult to regain completely because it is so easy to cheat! There is little motivation to fully use the hand and arm that is painful, especially if it happens to be your dominant hand and arm that is not sore. You can cheat even further because it is very seldom that you actually need the full range of arm movement to do something; it is quite possible to continue to use the arm within the narrow range of painless movement.

What will the result be? You end up with a frozen shoulder and marked limitation of movement which may have to be 'released' by manipulation under anaesthesia. This is an additional nuisance, painful, and requires another anaesthetic — not a good idea at all. It happened in my wife's case; we all thought she had done her exercises pretty well, but it had been within a limited range of relatively painless movement.

What exercises can be done?

Immediately post-op, during the first few days:

- gentle shoulder-rolling exercises;
- moving your arm gently away from the side where you have tucked it away like the broken wing of an injured bird;
- bringing the arm forward to 90 degrees, i.e., to shoulder height — no higher at this stage; and
- lifting the arm up sideways — again to shoulder height.

Once drains are out (see Figure 8.1): Increase your exercises slowly but surely. The aim is to have full range of movement re-established by four weeks after surgery, at the latest.

While exercising your muscles, exercise your mind. Look forward to your sessions: see the pain and discomfort as a temporary nuisance that will pass. Accept the challenge you have set yourself. Remember perseverance may not remove mountains, but it will allow you to scale them. There are always ten better things to do in life than give up.

Other forms of exercise

Walking

Go for walks, which can increase in both difficulty and duration as you get stronger. Walking and holding hands with someone and swinging that arm forwards and backwards helps. Get outside and explore nature: go for walks where you can enjoy peace and tranquillity, where you can smell pine trees or blossoms, where you can watch a meandering stream and where you can recharge your mental and emotional batteries. Nature is a great tonic and is free to all of us. Enjoy her healing and strengthening powers, her power to rejuvenate you, to help you see things in perspective and remind you of our fragile mortality.

Do not isolate yourself indoors. Do not stay locked in suburbia. Do not stay in a big city with all its impersonal noises and lack of involvement or commitment. Do not say, 'I don't want to try', even if walking was not something you did before having surgery. Now is a good time to start. While walking with your husband, lover, or a friend the gentle pace and motion of strolling allows for a comfortable relaxed atmosphere, and it is often a good time to openly and freely discuss intimate or closely-held fears and problems. It can be a very positive experience. Why not try it? If you prefer, and it is within reach, go and walk on the beach at sunset and allow the sound of the waves to calm your psyche and soul.

Jogging, cycling, swimming, and other non-contact sports

These are all beneficial and can be a new challenge to you. Take up something that you have never done before — persuade a friend or family member to start with you. This aspect is dealt with in more detail in Chapter 9, when we discuss healthy-living practices.

Getting back on the bicycle

As you sit in the dust when off your bike you fall
All you'll want to do is curl up into a small, grey ball
And say, 'To hell with it all — enough is enough!'
But remember that you are made of much much stronger staff
Because the lower you are, the less of the horizon will be seen
You won't know where you're going — only where you've been
Stand up again, climb back on your bike, and with a clearer head
Pedal strongly along the road that beckons ahead
There will be more hills that take a mighty effort to climb
But the view from the top will dry any tears that in your eyes do shine.

Effort requires character and character demands effort.

66 *I thought I was doing my arm exercises well when in fact I was doing them badly. I therefore had to have my frozen shoulder manipulated under anaesthetic.* **Jenny** 99

Chapter 9

The prospect of further treatment

Further treatment: What are the implications?

Before discussing specific methods of treatment, and looking at the circumstances that call for further treatment (see Figure 9.1), it is important to consider what the aims of the different modalities (forms) of treatment are.

Surgery

The basic aim of surgery is the removal of the cancer itself, with enough surrounding tissue to completely eradicate it. This is only potentially possible with a modified mastectomy, when all the breast tissue is removed. With any form of lumpectomy or partial mastectomy there is no guarantee that the whole cancer has been removed; nor is there any guarantee that there is not another focus of cancer within that breast which is as yet undetected. For this reason all forms of lumpectomy are followed by a course of radiation therapy to destroy any remaining cancer cells within the breast tissue and the 'bed' that the lump was removed from.

Surgery with gland removal

Here there are two approaches:

- Limited gland removal: Glands in the axilla drain upwards towards the inner armpit. It is therefore assumed that if the bottom glands are free then the upper ones must be too, and so some surgeons sample only the lowermost glands.
- Total gland removal: Other surgeons feel it is safer to take out all the glands right up into the apex (top) of the axilla. This is referred to as a modified radical mastectomy, as it is only the muscles of the chest wall that are not removed.

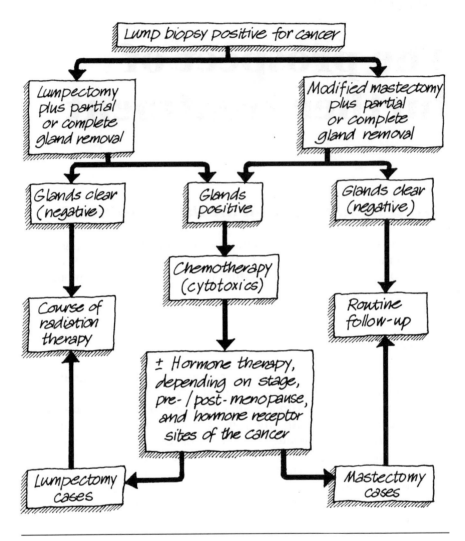

Figure 9.1 *Treatment strategies*

The advantage of this latter, total form of gland removal is that it is considered safer (perhaps only slightly so) to remove all the draining glands. The disadvantages are that there is a greater likelihood of lymphoedema (swelling due to lymph accumulation) in the arm, and there is also a greater risk of damage to a nerve that supplies sensation to the back of the shoulder and side of the chest. If this nerve is damaged you may be left with a numb area of skin with some parasthesia (increased burning/tingling sensation) in the adjacent area. This can improve markedly with time, but may only partially improve, as has occurred in my wife's case.

Why take out the glands?

This is now considered by almost all authorities to be mandatory. To remove the lump only and not to at least sample the lowermost glands is a potentially dangerous practice. If on histology the glands are free of evidence of cancer spread, then no further cytotoxic treatment is required. If you had any form of lumpectomy, then radiation therapy is commenced after two to four weeks of wound healing.

If the glands are positive (show evidence of cancer on histology), then further cytotoxic (chemotherapy) treatment is indicated. Such chemotherapy is indicated whether a lumpectomy or modified mastectomy has been performed. With a lumpectomy, further radiation therapy will then follow after cytotoxic therapy has been commenced — usually after a period of six weeks, though this varies considerably.

Cytotoxics (chemotherapy)

When cells multiply rapidly they are more susceptible to damage by agents which affect their basic function and metabolic pathways. This is how cytotoxics work. They can damage all cells, but fortunately do most damage to the cells multiplying fastest and in an uncontrolled way, such as cancer cells. These cells are selectively targeted no matter where they are 'hiding'. Different drugs work in different ways, and different cancers respond differently to different drug combinations. Because of this variability a combination of agents will often be used to achieve the maximum effect — almost like a 'therapy cocktail'. Depending on their type and form, these agents can either be given orally, by injection into muscle, or through a drip-line into a vein.

Radiation

Once again, radiation (small, invisible particle-bombardment of cells) can damage all cells, but cancer cells are more susceptible to damage than normal cells. Radiation therapy is directed at the target area using different techniques, for example directing the rays themselves (like aiming a gun), or by increasing local dosage by implanting radium needles (radio-active needles) in the target area.

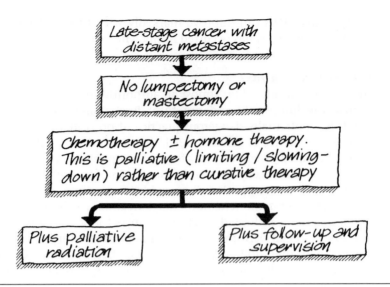

Figure 9.2 *Cancer that has spread*

Hormonal therapy

Using special histological identification techniques it can be determined whether or not a cancer has what is called hormone (oestrogen and/or progesterone) receptor sites. It has been shown that in patients who have cancer that has such receptor sites, additional hormonal therapy can further improve the prognosis (outlook). This outcome is also governed by other factors such as the stage of the cancer (stage I, II, III, or IV) and whether the patient is pre- or post-menopausal. This is a complex issue and it is best to let the experts advise what form of hormonal treatment, if any, is best suited to your particular situation and type of cancer.

The other role played by hormone therapy is in palliation (damping down or retarding but not curing). This occurs in the management of advanced disease that has spread beyond the local or regional area and where distant metastases are present. This form of therapy is one of limiting progression and reducing pain rather than being truly curative in nature.

You may have heard of people in the past having additional surgery to prevent or alter hormonal activity. Such surgery included removal of the ovaries (oophorectomy), removal of adrenals (adrenalectomy), or removal of the pituitary gland (hypophysectomy). With modern drugs such surgery is almost never indicated, except in occasional cases where oophorectomy may be recommended.

MASTECTOMY

Advantages	Disadvantages
Potentially cured with total removal of cancer and breast tissue	Frightening, painful, traumatic. Hospital admission
Reduces tumour mass (amount) so chemotherapy and body defence can destroy any remaining cancer in glands	Loss of breast and altered body image
Peace of mind at total breast-tissue removal	Need for reconstruction or external prosthesis
Remove glands for staging and determining need for further therapy	May develop lymphoedema (swelling) in arm on that side
Has been 'gold standard' of therapy for some time	Lumpectomy major alternative — there may be some confusion as to what is best for a particular patient

LUMPECTOMY

Advantages	Disadvantages
Potentially cured with total cancer removal	Still painful and traumatic, but less so than mastectomy. Hospital admission
Causes less damage to breast and therefore better body image	May leave behind some cancer or another site of cancer in the same breast
Quicker recovery period	Needs follow-up with radiation in all cases. Usually for up to 6 weeks
Glands — as for mastectomy	As for mastectomy
Better body image. Don't need reconstruction	Peace of mind may not be as complete
Retains breast and nipple sensation	Radiation and its local side-effects
Affords a choice and alternative to mastectomy	May cause problems deciding what is the right choice. Need for guidance and adequate information

Table 9.1 *The advantages and disadvantages of surgery*

Advantages	Disadvantages
Can destroy lurking cancer cells which cannot be seen, felt, or found in any other way	Treatment for up to six months after surgery, with nausea, hair loss, and marrow depression as possible side-effects
Can save your life and keep you well. Significant increase in disease-free survival	May need to be given intravenously, so must keep attending the hospital oncology department
Good results when cancer has spread to glands	Need further blood tests to monitor possible side-effects
Psychologically good additional support — knowing it can destroy unseen cancer cells	Emotional depression because of side-effects such as painful mouth, diarrhoea, fatigue, and vomiting in addition to those mentioned above
Can relieve pain and cause regression of large, distant metastases	Unlikely to cure large distant metastases completely
May prolong life in advanced cases	Seriously affects quality of such life
Can be stopped if a particular side-effect occurs	Dosage or frequency must be changed or same side-effect tends to recur
Other drugs are available to decrease side-effects such as nausea	Variable response in patients. Taking yet another drug!

There is a price to pay for success.

Table 9.2 *The advantages and disadvantages of chemotherapy*

How can you help yourself?

There can be little doubt that a healthy mind and positive attitude deserves to reside in a healthy body. There will be times that you will feel your body has in a way let you down, that it developed cancer and created an enormous problem in your life. However, you need to keep your body in the very best condition possible under the circumstances, so that it can work for you to the best of its ability.

Advantages	Disadvantages
Can destroy cancer cells left behind following lumpectomy	Cannot be used on its own to treat breast cancer (i.e., without surgery)
Can destroy unsuspected cancer in the area of breast tissue being irradiated	Can only be given after healing from surgery has occurred (after 4 weeks)
Can destroy cancer cells in draining glands	Cannot be given all at once. Must be given over ± 6 weeks. May cause increased lymphoedema
Can be given accurately and 'aimed' at specific high-risk areas	Must be given in a special unit. May be a frightening experience due to the machinery involved, etc.
Kills cancer cells	Kills/damages ordinary cells, leading to local pain and peeling skin. Possibility of increased cancer risk in some cells
Radioactive needles can be implanted in areas of high risk to increase the local effect	Slightly painful. Have to spend 3 or 4 days 'alone' while the radium works
Can be given to specific area before reconstruction	May cause local thickening and tightness of the skin and scarring of the chest wall, making reconstruction more difficult
Not painful while being given	Local pain of skin, breast, or chest wall, and may 'burn', the skin as an after-effect
Can be aimed at a specific secondary to control pain-pressure effects	Cannot totally cure or kill a large mass of cancer such as a large secondary which is causing symptoms

A powerful 'ray-gun' to defend yourself with

Table 9.3 *The advantages and disadvantages of radiotherapy*

Advantages	Disadvantages
Can be given in addition to all other forms of therapy	Most effective in certain types of cancer rich with 'receptor' sites
Can render further surgery unnecessary, such as removal of adrenal glands or ovaries	May cause thinning of the bones (osteoporosis) or long-term heart disease
Very effective in pain-control of distant metastases	Only works for some patients
Newer agents have minimal side-effects	Research necessary to determine best combinations of therapy
Can in some cases improve the results of chemotherapy (called hormonal synchronization)	Needs specialist knowledge and skills to use combination most effectively
Less side-effects than chemotherapy — can be used sequentially (following each other)	Tends to hold cancer in check or cause some regression. Usually not curative by itself
More effective in post-menopausal women	Less effective in pre-menopausal women
Decreases recurrence rate and improves 5-year survival rate	Must be given for a long time. May cause weight gain, depression, hot flushes, nausea, and sweating

Some hormones switch cancer on; others switch it off.

Table 9.4 *The advantages and disadvantages of hormone therapy*

Interesting research studies have been done regarding the effects on the body's defence mechanisms of exercise and staying fit. It is clear that staying fit and exercising (sometimes difficult to maintain, depending on treatment and side-effects) has a beneficial effect on the body's immune system, so exercise falls into a 'total care' bracket.

Other benefits to be derived from exercise include an impressive improvement of over 20% in work capacity in those exercising compared to those not exercising, and considerably less weakening and thinning of the bones (osteoporosis). Other advantages of any good programme of exercise include improved heart function and endurance, muscle strength, flexibility, reduced body fat, improved blood fat (lipid profile — cholesterol and triglycerides), and an improved psychological profile. With all this for it, what is there against it? Nothing. It does at first take will-power, determination, and organization of your life, but it should become part of your new way of living.

A healthy mind and attitude

What makes life dreary is lack of motive. So create new challenges — mental or physical — and then tackle them with enthusiasm and without delay. Once you have been diagnosed positive for breast cancer, the first challenges may well be forced on you as you are called to respond to the outcomes of your therapy, which can be pretty tough-going.

But what about after this? It may help to remember that difficulties are the normal thing in every worthwhile life; it's just that some people get more than their fair share of problems. The well-known quotation, 'Grant me the strength to change the things I can, to accept the things I cannot change, and the wisdom to know the difference' certainly applies to anyone with breast cancer. Although you may never learn to completely accept breast cancer, you may well discipline yourself so that you can live with it in a way that is not crippling to you as an individual with your own dreams, hopes, intentions, and goals.

Your mind, like your body, needs exercise. It can be kept active and supple by using it to its fullest capacity. There are 'filing cabinets' in your mind that probably have not been opened in years, and yet they are full of invaluable facts and information, forgotten dreams and precious ambitions. Open the filing cabinets! Get on and tackle your almost-forgotten dreams or ambitions — it is not too late. One is never too old to feel young: old age is related much more to a loss of interest than to your age in years. This is a good time to resurrect unfulfilled dreams and ambitions and, with new priorities in your life, to do something about them. You are on a voyage of rediscovery.

'But what if I make a mistake?' I can hear you asking. 'What if I can't tackle what I set out to do? What if I don't succeed in what I try to do?' Firstly, you can turn back if you find you are on the wrong road. It may mean that it takes a little longer to get onto the right one, but you can retrace your steps. Secondly, you are never the poorer for having tried. You are living a dreary life if your only aim is to stand still! Someone who is an optimist is usually a success, because their mind is not occupied with reasons why a thing *cannot* be done.

A healthy body

Confidence is the companion of success. One way to improve your confidence is to get your body into shape. Clearly this depends on your age, physical ability, individual situation, and so on, but I am willing to bet that each and every one of you can get yourself into better shape than you are in now.

Start by getting up earlier: by rising an hour earlier every day you gain almost a whole extra 'doing day' per week. Not only that, but an hour in the morning is worth two in the evening. If possible, sit where you can watch the sun rising to herald the new day; you can almost hear the trumpets of life if you close your eyes and listen carefully. My wife adores the 'hours of long shadows' (both morning and evening), when the colours are muted and the plants and trees lose their clear-cut margins. It is as if your soul is given a vigorous pummelling, told to get itself on parade, brace itself — life is on the move.

'Between the great things we believe we cannot do and the small things we will not do, lies the danger that we will do nothing.' So start small: go for walks, even take up gentle jogging or cycling, get a small exercise trampolene at home, and do a series of physical exercises for arm and chest muscles using small, light-weight dumbells. Work your way up gently and steadily, but start! There are many people — doctors, physios, and gym trainers — who can give you professional help and guidance and advise on a graded, increasing schedule of exercise.

The aims are to increase your cardiovascular endurance, to improve your muscle tone and strength, and to improve flexibility, movement, and posture. Such a programme should include the following ingredients, can be done at home or at a health club or gymnasium, and should be done at least twice a week.

Phase one: Warm-up exercise on an exercise bicycle, or jogging trampolene, or treadmill

Phase two: Stretching movements to increase flexibility and isometric-type exercises (using your muscle contractions to work against and tone other muscles)

Phase three: Increasing your heart rate and maintaining it there by doing aerobic exercises on a bicycle, treadmill, trampolene or in an aerobics class

Phase four: Muscle stengthening and conditioning using light weights with rapid, repetitive types of circuit exercise

Phase five: Endurance-type exercise such as using a rowing machine

Phase six: Cooling-down exercises: slower movement, stretching, and recovering. Have a sauna and shower. Relax and feel good. Enjoy the sense of achievement even if you are tired.

In addition to such a programme you should walk, jog, cycle, or swim three times a week. 'Phew!' I can just hear you say, 'This guy has gone crazy — I can't do that'. Well I beg to differ: I know you can. But the way to do it is to start slowly, gain strength and confidence, and end up strong (in so many ways, because being physically fit will make you emotionally stronger and mentally more alert).

Healthy eating and drinking

In Afrikaans there is the little word 'te'. It is like the English word 'too', but somehow much more descriptive and expressive. Much like the English 'too', when 'te' is used it usually indicates an unhealthy, unhappy, uncomfortable, or unpleasant situation — 'too' little, 'too' much, 'too' hard, 'too' soft, and so on — and usually indicates that something is potentially wrong one way or another. How does this relate to healthy eating? A balanced diet must not be too strict, too lenient, too little, too much, too fat, too lean, too big, or too small. The following are good general guidelines:

- Reduce your total fat consumption, and particularly saturated fat and cholesterol, mainly through reducing fatty meats and high-fat dairy products.
- Increase your intake of whole-grain cereals and bread, fibre, pasta, peas, and beans.
- Increase your intake of fresh fruit and vegetables of all sorts.
- Eat fish instead of meat or high-fat dairy products.
- Try to avoid artificial flavourings, colourings, salt, and processed foods.

As regards drinking, moderation is again the key word. Drinking plays an important role in our health and in social interaction. 'Too much' tea, coffee, full-cream milk, alcohol, carbonated drink, fruit juice (or even water!) can have potentially harmful side-effects. As with diet, a balanced fluid intake — without necessarily excluding any drink in particular — is unlikely to cause harm. No specific drinks have been scientifically linked to the development of breast cancer, but many of the components used in drinks do have significant known side-effects. These include tannin and caffeine in tea, caffeine in coffee and coke, fats in milk, alcohol in all alcoholic drinks, sugar in carbonated drinks, and the high electrolyte content of some fruit juices and health drinks. Even excessive water-drinking can cause electrolyte disturbances in the body.

Smoking

While smoking as such has not been directly linked to causing breast cancer, it has so many other potentially lethal or debilitating side-effects (lung cancer, chronic respiratory disease, increased risk of coronary heart disease, hypertension (high blood pressure), stroke, and circulatory problems) that health-wise it rates as one of the most dangerous habits. If you smoke, you are much more likely to die from one of its side-effects than you are to die from breast cancer, which is a sobering thought.

Healthy loving

To love and to be loved are among the greatest joys of life. Loving takes many forms: the protective love of a parent, the caring, concerned love of a partner, and the warm and enhancing love of a good friend. One common denominator in all loving relationships is that of really caring. Another is the act of giving. What we give to others in life we receive from; what we share with others will continue to increase and multiply, but what we keep to ourselves is lost forever once we are gone. Giving is not merely physical, financial, or material; giving includes encouragement, understanding, support, empathy, and sacrifice.

Sexual relationships

The other aspect of love in a relationship may be the physical expression of love-making. It can take many forms, and has many important ingredients that comprise what may seem to be a simple, basic act. Love-making contains aspects of tenderness, mutual pleasure, sharing, excitement, and emotional relief, with mental relaxation far beyond the pure sexual satisfaction which is so often focused on. It can be participated in in many ways besides the final common pathway of actual physical intercourse.

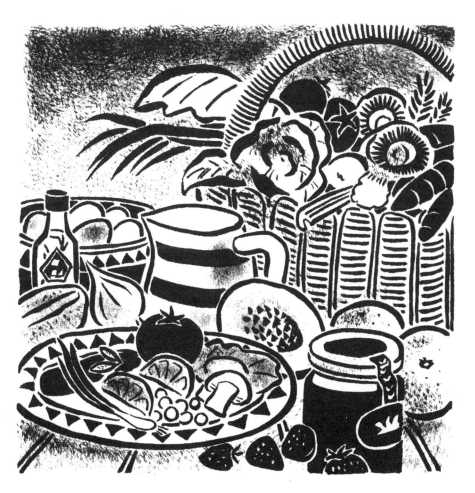

Minds and attitudes are crucial in giving expression to a relaxed and enjoyable natural act. Fear, anxiety, or apprehension can prove to be as much a damper to the small flame of early arousal as can a bucket of water to a match flame. If the flame goes out or the match does not strike at all there will be no ensuing fire of passion to warm the soul and comfort the mind.

Confidence

Confidence in your own sexuality is of paramount importance in this process. Confidence in turn comes from belief in yourself, your relationship, your ability, and your own body image. Breast cancer can have a profound effect on all these aspects and thereby can become an obstacle to achieving a return to your previous love-making pattern, let alone trying to improve it.

An obstacle is anything which stands in the way, a hindrance, or an obstruction. If you know it is going to be there, one way of overcoming it may be to make plans to achieve the same destination via a different route. Secondly, when you do come across an obstacle, plans can and must be made to remove it from the path or to clamber over or round it as you continue on your way. It must not be allowed to stop you.

Breast cancer often occurs at a stage in life when bodies are not as firm or strong as they were, when sexual activity was already declining, and when relationships are moving into a comfortable form of companionship rather than being strongly physical. To have breast cancer superimposed on this can be potentially disastrous to a couple's sex-life. Active, positive steps must be taken to ensure that you do not withdraw into a cocoon of sexual isolation.

The first step to take is to resume your previous role as wife and/or lover, and friend. The ultimate aim is to improve your relationship beyond this point, but the first goal is to be as you were before. This is not always easy. Take the same care with your appearance and the way you dress. The extent to which this instils confidence will vary a lot from one woman to another. Do not move into the 'baggy look': in the early stages, while there is still discomfort, before a prosthesis has been fitted or reconstruction has been done, loose, comfortable tops are fine, but they must not become a shield behind which you continue to try to hide your 'deformity'. Be comfortable, yes, but not impersonal and sexless! Re-establishing confidence in your femininity is a good basis for taking further steps into sexual security and growth.

In each particular relationship there will be specific factors which will be more pertinent than others. These include personality, beliefs, customs, attitudes, upbringing, concepts, openness, degree of anxiety, and interpersonal communication skills. I cannot offer further specific guidance, as each case is different, but the following thoughts with regard to reconstruction, honesty, and shyness may be helpful.

Reconstruction

I am strongly in favour of reconstruction. For almost every woman who has had a mastectomy it is the biggest single boost to morale and confidence in her femininity, and there is little to compare with it for lasting effect. Total sexual responsiveness, including the degree and length of arousal, is usually improved following reconstruction. This works through the complex, interconnected pathways of the mind and body rather than the physical stimulating pathways from the reconstructed breast (physical sensation in the reconstructed breast tends to remain minimal).

Honesty

You and your partner must pluck up the courage to discuss openly your fears, feelings, and frustrations. This is easier said than done, but if you do start — even timidly — to discuss such feelings, you will be amazed how much easier it becomes to discuss them in more depth. The man has a crucial role to play: he must express his desire for you through both attitude and action. In many situations he will show himself to be more tender than before, more caring in his attentions to your needs, and more concerned as to your welfare. There is nothing quite so sobering as having to face the possibility of losing the one you love (one who perhaps you were taking just a little bit for granted), the one who you cannot imagine yourself living without. Cancer is a frightening and serious diagnosis, and puts values in life in perspective very rapidly. Many partners find that love-making becomes more gentle and meaningful, has a larger emotional element, and expresses more honest appreciation for each other than tended to happen before.

Don't be shy

You must not be shy. The first step is to brace yourself and be determined not to alter any previous behaviour patterns. Many women who used to undress totally comfortably in front of their partners now want to do so in privacy; lights that used to be left on are now switched off; baths and showers that used to be taken together are now avoided at all costs. No! No! No! This must not be allowed to happen. The more you 'hide it' the more 'exposed' the problem becomes. Encourage your husband or partner to see, feel, and kiss the breast after lumpectomy, the scarred area after mastectomy, and the reconstructed breast when it has been done. This takes a lot of guts on your part, and he may be even more unsure of himself than you are. You may have to take a leading role in this regard. Proceed slowly and gently, but be sure to proceed — do not regress.

Failed relationships

You hear many stories of relationships coming apart because the man in the couple could not handle it, could not face it, could not overcome the loss of a breast in the woman he 'loved'. What a lot of nonsense! Such relationships were doomed to fail anyway — it was just a matter of time. He would have packed his bags sometime in the future when a crisis occurred which required some courage, fortitude and character on his part. Sadly, while this is true, the effect of such a loss on the confidence and recovery of the person who has had the mastectomy can be a major negative one. It does not help her to know that he lacked basic moral fibre, did not have the required guts and courage, and did not truly love her.

How can a man compare loving a person and regaining something so precious in his life with the relatively small problem of her losing a breast? It makes no sense at all. Getting losses and gains in perspective is essential.

Expectations

It would be unfair on yourself to expect or attempt a major change in your basic character make-up. I am therefore not suggesting for a moment that if you are a shy, introverted, and conservative person you can suddenly turn into an outgoing, openly demonstrative, relaxed-about-physical-exposure type of individual. Such a metamorphosis is highly unlikely! But what must not be allowed to happen is you becoming more shy, introverted, and conservative than before. Use this new situation as a challenge to grow in your loving and your sex-life. Devise new and interesting ways of being together — bathing by candlelight, for instance — explore different forms and emphases in love-making, and improve the quality of togetherness time. With a positive mind and attitude you could well gain more in your relationship than you have lost. Try it.

It has been said that women are the most remarkable foreigners with whom men come into contact. A man will always only partly understand you, always have only partial insight into how you function, your complexities, and your sense of values, and only partly be able to share your innermost feelings. This 'partly' can be a little 'partly' or a considerable 'partly'. With your help and encouragement and with his involvement and interest it must become a considerable 'partly'. The world is full of willing people — some willing to try, the others willing to let them. In this instance you must both be triers!

Stay physical

66 *I was so grateful that I did not need further treatment and did not have to face the ordeal of losing my hair. I feel so sorry for women who have the trauma of losing their hair as well as having to lose a breast, which is shock enough.*
Jenny   **99**

> **"** *One of my favourite sayings, from Winston Abbot, is that it is often not easy to remember that in the fading light of day ... the shadows always point towards the dawn.*
> **Jenny** **"**

Chapter 10

Reconstruction

Complexities involved and personal attitudes

Reconstruction is a subject which triggers many emotions, much discussion, and many different approaches depending on whether lay, professional, conservative, radical, male, or female points of view are taken into account. It is also an extremely personal decision. Table 10.1. demonstrates some of the differences in women's attitudes to reconstruction.

It must be stressed that these attitudes are never an entirely black or white, clear-cut affair: there is always a degree of ambivalence which is often either not admitted to or not even recognized.

A *man's point of view*

Considering all the variable personal needs, expectations, and fears outlined in Table 10.1, it is abundantly clear that one course cannot serve all these personal needs. All I can do, therefore, is give my point of view and inform you of the options open to you. Once you know what research and psychological assessment profiles have revealed, the final, informed decision is up to you.

My point of view is obviously that of a male and is therefore unquestionably biased. I sincerely believe that virtually all women regardless (to a point) of age will benefit from reconstruction. The benefit for most is tremendous; considerable for others; moderate for a small number; and almost never insignificant. That is a pretty sweeping statement, and may well be criticized by women who have opted or who will opt not to have reconstruction done, and who have coped or will cope quite adequately.

For reconstruction	Against reconstruction
Body image is important and breasts are an important part of body image	Body image is important but breasts are not an important part of body image
Completeness of body image	Body image is not important
Not too old to worry about body image	Too old to mind about it
Love me and my breasts	Love me — not my breasts
Breasts are important in my sexuality and my life	Breasts and/or sexuality are not important in my life
Reconstruction more comfortable to handle and live with than a prosthesis	Prosthesis perfectly adequate, or don't even need a prosthesis as I don't mind being lop-sided and I love my body as it is
Will gain in overall confidence	Will not affect overall confidence
Will be more comfortable with my partner	Will not be more comfortable with my partner
Will help my husband or partner to accept me	Will not help my husband or partner to accept me
No fears regarding long-term problems with silicone-bag implants	Many fears regarding long-term problems with silicone-bag implants
Prepared to accept more surgery	Will not accept more surgery
Will not influence further cancer development	Might influence further cancer development

Table 10.1 *Pros and cons of reconstruction*

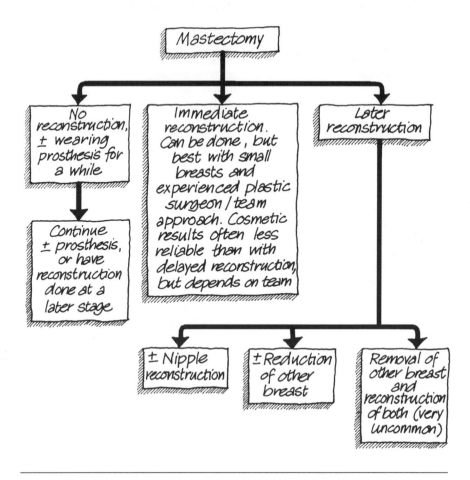

Figure 10.1 *Possible strategies for reconstruction after mastectomy*

Only you can determine what is best for you. I question whether you might not be better-off with a reconstruction, but experience has left me with a strong personal bias in its favour.

Backing up this attitude

In the past (as recently as ten years ago), reconstruction was offered to women only if it was felt that they could not cope emotionally with their changed body image. It was given to them as a kind of psychological crutch. It was wrongly assumed that such women were less well-adjusted than those who could cope with their disfigurement and live with their amputation with appropriate resignation. Research has shown this to be totally wrong! The woman who seeks reconstruction is exhibiting positive coping and problem-solving manoeuvres; it is an appropriate response for a well-adjusted woman, not a discontented, neurotic reaction. How things can change! What motivates such women is the need to feel whole again, to get rid of an external prosthesis and to have a better body image. As reconstruction techniques have improved, and as doctors' attitudes as to who needs or benefits from reconstruction have changed considerably, so reconstruction is becoming the norm.

Sexual responsiveness and reconstruction

Research has demonstrated that breast reconstruction increases sexual responsiveness. This in all likelihood occurs largely through an improvement in a woman's sense of her own physical attractiveness, which is linked to her sexual responsiveness. But there is much more to this complex issue than that: studies show women who have had breast reconstruction to be more readily sexually aroused than a non-reconstructed control group. This may be linked to overt or covert anxiety in the women who have not had reconstruction. Such anxiety gets transmitted into a negative preoccupation with their physical appearance. This makes it hard to 'let go' and enjoy love-making and the pleasures of the moment, and concentrates their attention on a negative aspect rather than a positive one.

Studies have also confirmed that there were differences not only in the time taken to be aroused, but also in the magnitude of sexual excitement experienced.

While the reconstructed breast itself does not really serve as an erotic zone, the complexity of sexual response is such that differences were even shown between two groups of women who had had reconstruction with or without a nipple. The only way to explain such a difference is the sense of completeness or wholeness in the nipple-reconstructed group — we are back to the power of the mind again!

Is this true for everyone?

The answer is clearly no. Sexual activity, drive, and degree of arousal are subject to many influencing factors, not least of all age. Some people are sexually active longer into their later years than others. Your sex-life is so personal and individual that for some women, especially with the right partner, reconstruction is not necessary. In fact there is evidence that love-making can become more meaningful, be more tender, and express more feeling once you are much more aware of the precious gift of life and of the slender and tenuous thread of human mortality.

So the issue of reconstruction remains complex, personal, and is governed by individual beliefs and attitudes. I would, however, encourage you to make full enquiries about what is available to you, to look at it from all angles, and to weigh up pros and cons before accepting or discarding it.

What can be done and when?

The three main options open to you are shown in Figure 10.1, but it is not quite as clear-cut as this. You will need to be advised by your surgeon and perhaps by the plastic surgeon he or she works with. In many cases they have developed and established a course of action which results in what they consider to be the best outcome for the patient (and thus also for them). They may, however be somewhat conservative and set in their ways, and may take the course that is more convenient for them without considering the emotional make-up and needs of individual patients as regards timing of the reconstruction.

Indications for immediate reconstruction

Immediate reconstruction requires a surgical team capable of, and comfortable with, performing such immediate surgery, so you will have to research this prerequisite before considering the option. Some surgical teams will not perform immediate reconstruction, for various reasons, but this seems to be changing. Large breasts are an adverse factor, as either reduction of the other breast or the amount of skin available for reconstruction complicates the issue.

Patients who are good candidates psychologically for immediate reconstruction include women who:
- are extremely breast-orientated and who see this as synonymous with their self-worth;
- are very resistant to having a mastectomy unless intra-operative repair is an option;
- are well-read, fully informed, and who believe implicitly that the benefits outweigh the risks;

- are young and assertive, and for whom the wearing of a prosthesis is totally out of keeping with their life-style;
- have strong negative images of mastectomy without reconstruction, either because of an actual experience with a relative or friend, or from reading magazine articles on the subject;
- have a cancer-phobia about the remaining breast and want to lessen the trauma of a prophylactic mastectomy with a simultaneous reconstruction.

Delayed reconstruction

In this course of action reconstruction is delayed for at least three months to allow all swelling to disappear and primary healing to occur. Delay may be up to six months to allow for the completion of chemotherapy or radiation treatment. Different techniques are then used by different surgeons, and depend on a number of factors, of which two are major:
- the size of the silicone bag to be inserted in order to match the other breast; and
- the amount of strength and the degree of 'tightness' of the chest wall as regards allowing for the implantation of the prosthesis under the chest muscles.

If the remaining breast is very large, a breast reduction may need to be done simultaneously on that side. Even so, a two-stage surgical approach may still be necessary: a smaller bag is implanted initially, allowed to stretch the tissue and skin over a period of weeks, and then as a second stage this first bag is removed and a larger one inserted. There are also bags which can be placed under the skin and which can then be systematically 'blown up' with fluid, causing a steady pressure stretch of the skin until enough stretch is achieved to enable the silicone prosthesis to be inserted comfortably.

I have concentrated on reconstruction techniques which use silicone-bag implants as these are by far the commonest form used for reconstruction. There are many other techniques available where the fat and skin of the patient is used to create the breast mound. Details of procedures can be given to you by a plastic surgeon who uses such techniques.

Having more surgery after healing from your mastectomy is clearly a major stumbling block, and often frightens off the wary, weary, or worried patient. My personal feeling (easy once again for me to say) is that what is gained by going through the additional trauma of more surgery and expense far outweighs what is lost by not having it done. The additional sacrifice will be worth it once it is all over.

Realistic expectations of the end result

The term 'breast reconstruction' is perhaps unfortunate, as it is in fact a misnomer. If you expect to get back a breast similar to the one you lost, you will be disappointed. No matter how brilliant, experienced, or determined your plastic/reconstruction surgeon may be, he cannot work miracles — wonders yes, miracles no. Size, shape, consistency, and sensation will all be different, even if only slightly so, in all women. Do not start off with unrealistic expectations, or you are sure to be unhappy with the result. When compared with a flat chest wall, the creation of a silicone breast-mound is a 100% improvement. However, when compared to a normal breast it will only be 60–70% as cosmetically effective. It will mean a better body image, easier wearing of clothing, body-hugging tops or bathing costumes. It will be much easier to adapt to emotionally than having no breast at all, and will make nudity more comfortable — but it will still be different. You will have to adjust to and learn to live with the reconstruction. A better term would be 'the creation of a breast mound'. You must be a realist in this regard.

With or without a nipple?

Some, probably most, plastic surgeons do not reconstruct a nipple during the initial breast reconstruction, as the scar often stretches across the breast and creates nipple-positioning problems. Nipple reconstruction is therefore usually done after healing has occurred. By now you are tired of surgical procedures. Is it worth it? Many women opt not to have it done and are 'perfectly happy'. It does leave you with a small problem with wearing modern T-shirts, bikinis, bathing costumes, bras and clinging tops where the missing nipple-bulge could be obvious and therefore restrict your clothing choice to some extent. Nipples are now quite simply created by a so-called 'purse string' suture (stitch) being used to gather together a button (nubbin) of skin. The areola (pigmented area around a normal nipple) is then simply tattooed on around the purse-string button. This is simple, very effective, and looks almost like the real thing. It is not very uncomfortable to have done, and research shows that this degree of completeness further enhances body image, femininity, and sexuality. At the very least it is worth considering seriously whether or not to have it done.

What's all the fuss about silicone?

It is important that the silicone issue be put in perspective, as the media has given it a lot of dramatic headline exposure. Many of the original so-called complications or disasters linked to silicone stem from the era when it was injected directly into breast tissue to augment what nature provided in the first place. Nature does not like foreign material, even relatively inert material such as silicone, to be injected directly into tissue. As part of the body's healing process irritation is then expressed either in the form of a local inflammatory response or with fibrosis and scarring, thereby causing dimpling or deformity of the breast contour. There is no statistical proof whatsoever in these cases that there is an increased risk of cancer which would not have occurred anyway — merely assumptions made without supportive evidence and then often dramatized by the media.

What about silicone-bag implants?

These must be from a reliable source and of the highest quality. There are unscrupulous manufacturers who produce a cheap-and-nasty product which has been known to leak. Any reputable surgeon will always ensure that he uses the very best quality of silicone-bag prosthesis available; it is very much in the surgeon's own interest to do so as well as the patient's. Under no circumstances will such silicone bag implants cause further cancer to occur.

What can go wrong?
- When the bag is inserted a haematoma (blood clot) may form at the site of insertion and need to be drained. In a very small percentage of women the wound may become infected.
- The prosthesis is slipped into a pocket created behind the big chest muscle (pectoralis major). With arm movement and keeping the bag mobile this pocket will eventually form a fibrous capsule (this is a natural reaction of the body to 'wall it off'). The fibrous capsule may, however, become too tight as the body 'overreacts', and is then called a capsular contracture. This leads to a much less mobile prosthesis and a 'tight' breast mound.

  Unfortunately this may occur in up to 25% of patients. While it is annoying, irritating, and disappointing, it is fixable.

The capsule can be split (capsulectomy) and another silicone bag inserted.

You may well feel that there is no direct, uncomplicated, and straight-forward route in breast-cancer treatment. It is certainly a diagnosis that presents a lot of anxiety-provoking possibilities, difficult and complex decisions, and seemingly unjust side-effects or complications. The final take-home message is that despite all this you *can* win through and continue with a meaningful, productive, and fulfilling life in all respects.

What can I do after a reconstruction?

Simply put: almost everything you wish to do and that you were previously capable of doing (and more!). You can run, hop, cycle, swim, climb, walk, dance, play golf, tennis, squash, horse-ride, bird-watch, ski, jump, row, shoot, paddle, fly, or just sit and think about doing all these things.

You cannot play rugby, American football, or take part in all-in wrestling (or any other major bodily-contact sport — except love-making of course). Perhaps also give bungee jumping a miss!

What about breast reduction?

To have excessively large breasts reduced in size is an option that is available to women who feel very uncomfortable (often both physic-ally and mentally) about their excessively large breasts. This anxiety occurs particularly in short women whose very large breasts contrast starkly with their lack of height and prove especially embarrassing. The anxiety may result from comments being passed or may be of purely physical origin due to the breasts themselves impeding com-fortable everyday living. Large breasts can prevent the achievement of maximum potential in a particular sport such as gymnastics, ath-letics, or long-distance running, which can be an additional consid-eration for breast reduction. Often more than one factor influences the decision.

Breast reduction has no effect on the incidence of breast cancer, and certainly does not cause it. For women still worried about silicone, no silicone is used in breast reduction surgery. In fact the size reduction will allow for better assessment of the remaining breast tissue in the future, both by palpation and mammography, thereby facilitating the earlier detection of any abnormality such as breast cancer.

The skill of the plastic surgeon is of the utmost importance as regards the final cosmetic outcome. In some cases the nipple will need to be repositioned, with consequent loss of some sensation in that area.

Breast reduction surgery can dramatically improve a woman's body image, which will in turn affect other aspects such as self-confidence, personality, and ability. It is clearly a very personal decision, but it is important that doctors do not try to dissuade or discourage once such a decision has been made by a woman with excessively large breasts. Comments such as, 'Oh, your breasts aren't that big!' are ill-judged and have no place in giving guidance. What the *patient* feels, or is embarrassed or incapacitated by is what counts.

Long-term benefit is also an important consideration. The sheer weight of very large breasts can cause poor posture and back problems, and deep furrows will often form on the shoulders from constant bra-strap pressure. Most of these problems can be avoided by early reduction of the breast-weight.

For the right women it is the correct procedure, and is like lifting a weight off their shoulders — both literally and figuratively.

Reduction after mastectomy

Reduction of the remaining breast after a mastectomy may be indicated to simplify reconstruction. If the remaining breast is very large, it is impossible to match it with an equally large silicone-bag implant. This therefore requires a 'balancing' reduction in size. It is often done at the same time as the reconstruction on the other side, but it may require a two-stage procedure: reduction of the remaining breast first, followed by a reconstruction later to match the reduced breast.

The wearing of a prosthesis

If an immediate reconstruction was not done, or you are still deciding whether to have one done, or you have decided against reconstruction, then you will probably want a prosthesis. They are only available through certain stockists, and the Cancer Association or the Breast Cancer Clinic at the hospital in your area will be able to supply addresses. They vary in type and quality. A good one in a specialized rubber compound will cost between R300 and R500. Their lifespan is limited to three to four years, beyond which they tend to perish. Many patients choose to make their own padded cup which fits inside the bra, using cotton wool or other padding material. Birdseed bags which were used previously had the draw-back of weight but did mould well. They are no longer very popular.

Up to 50% of women, especially in the older age group, will decide against reconstruction. Without being too persistent I would still encourage you to reconsider such a decision.

> **❝** *I am so proud of my reconstruction, and even now, seven years later, I still marvel at how clever it all is. It isn't exactly like the other side, but then it can't be. It has played a major role in me being my normal self and I love it as I would an adopted child!* **Jenny** **❞**

Chapter 11

The roles that people play

The man's role

Many of the ways in which a man can offer support to help his partner overcome breast cancer have already been dealt with in different sections of this book. Let us recap some of these and look a little more closely at the man's role. Many well-ingrained expectations govern most men's behaviour: don't show emotion; keep a stiff upper lip; don't be a cry-baby; don't be a weakling; put on a brave face; don't be a sissy. Statements such as, 'It's human to show emotion; big men can and do cry; crying is a sign of caring and not of weakness; showing emotion is natural in a complete man' somehow don't convince most men that it really is acceptable to become emotionally involved, that it is OK to care enough to cry. Many men were brought up believing that 'big boys don't cry', and have great difficulty in showing that in fact they do care, or in expressing it without feeling terribly awkward. They are conditioned to be the provider, the defender of the family, and the one who you can depend and lean on.

When a man is threatened with losing the most precious person in his life through breast cancer and at the same time is expected to console her about the loss of a breast, he is sometimes not sure what to do. Some may try the tough, macho image and bluster their way through, giving the occasional pat on the back and saying, 'Keep it up, you are doing a great job!' Others may not be sure what to do or say, and as a result will withdraw and distance themselves from the whole scene — they are there in person but not there in being, and tend to keep themselves busily occupied doing male things. On the other hand, some men will be able to express their love and concern for their wife or partner, and are able to raise the curtain on the stage of their emotions. Such men can hug, hold, and comfort you, and may even be capable of weeping with you.

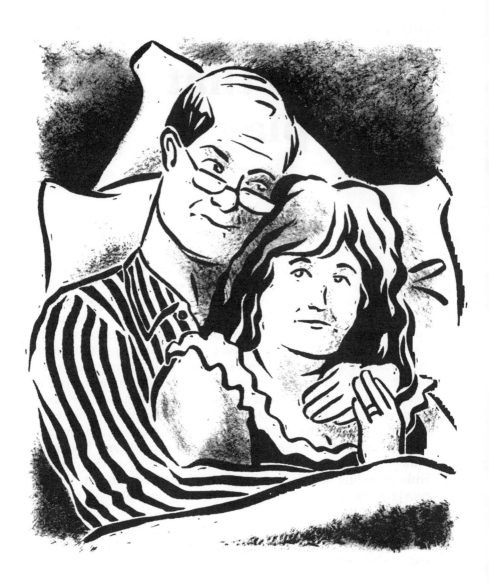

You will probably know better than anyone what the man in your life is like. You are often going to have to be the puppeteer. You must pull the right strings in order to get the most out of him. Show him that you want his involvement and encourage it. Let him understand that decisions should be made together, with dual responsibility and involvement; that this is not a one-woman show but a partnership; that while his role can still be one of being 'tough and strong', it must also be one of involvement and expressing his inner feelings.

There are many ways of consoling someone. All the senses can be used: through sight you can see his loving reaction and that he truly cares; through hearing you can be told in so many ways about what he feels and fears; through the sense of touch you can be tightly embraced, hugged, or just have your hand held during the difficult explanatory discussions and decision-making phases. A protective arm around you during those dark hours at night when your imagination seems to go into overdrive can be incredibly comforting. In all these ways a man is still fulfilling his protective role.

Even through the sense of smell you can be comforted — the smell of your favourite flowers or of a special perfume that he bought for you can be a form of solace. Wearing his favourite perfume while in hospital before and after surgery will be a reminder of him and make him seem closer when he is not there.

Most men do care deeply. Most would like to show that they care, but often do not know how to — how not to lose face and how to appear strong yet supportive is often a dilemma. With understanding on your part, and by gently coaxing and leading, you may well reach a stage where you gain the emotional and physical support you need while he still feels important and valued. It is often largely a matter of role-play which must be modified according to the particular needs of the two principal players involved. They represent a partnership which must now continue to grow and mature through a process of stress and emotional strife. Relationships often gain in stature and improve in quality under such circumstances.

Men do care but may not know how to show it.

66 *Our relationship, which was already very special, has become even better. Close has become closer. I have John to thank for my life.* **Jenny** 99

66 *Nothing is more sobering than becoming aware that you could lose someone you love when such an event was something you had never considered at this stage of your life.* **John** 99

Maintaining a sense of humour

There are some very serious situations in life where humour has no place, especially during the early stages of adjustment to the diagnosis of breast cancer. But there are other times where it does have a role to play. The ability to laugh at yourself or at the situation you find yourself in is often a tonic to the soul. This is not always easy to do, but it is important. I remember well a very brave young doctor called Barbara, who lost an arm and a leg in a shark attack on our dangerous east coast. With great guts and determination she returned after a year, fitted with an artificial leg and arm, to complete her housemanship. She had also taught herself to write with the other hand in less than a year. Despite her handicap she managed admirably and we (the other housemen/interns) would often allow her to struggle on until she had succeeded in a particular procedure or job she was trying to carry out. Late one night, at the end of a long day of being on call, she remarked to us that the bottom of her foot was itching and burning something terrible. The chorus of replies from the other assembled housemen was immediately, 'Which one?'. We all, including Barbara, had a good laugh and it was indicative of a form of close camaraderie. Being able to joke about her handicap was an expression of our acceptance and understanding of her problems, and was neither callous nor unfeeling.

Similarly, after having a mastectomy there can be light-hearted remarks made between people who love one another which help to ease discomfort, reveal full acceptance, and actually are an expression of love. Remarks by the man such as, 'Surely there are easier ways to lose weight?' or, 'I was spoilt with two, but one is plenty for me', or, 'You somehow look different — have you had your hair done?' can all go a long way towards lessening tension and improving acceptance. The humorous approach only works for some people, and the timing is of course all-important. In our case my wife became known as 'The Bionic Woman — a woman for all seasons', because the reconstructed breast with the silicone implant behind the muscle is considerably cooler to the touch than the normal one — so a warm breast for winter and a cool one for summer — a woman for all seasons!

Another interesting approach was to look on the reconstructed breast as if you had an 'adopted child' who needed as much care and attention (if not more) than the original 'child'. A bit like non-identical twins, each with their own specific characteristics but both needing to be taken note of and requiring individual attention.

If humour seems too frivolous for your situation or feels awkward, then do not use it. But it must be replaced with total honesty and complete frankness. Through open and honest discussion problems are solved rather than created. Awareness of someone's feelings allows behaviour modification to occur. Little progress can be made in improving understanding between individuals until it is known where each stands on a particular issue. This provides a point of reference, a yardstick against which to measure appropriate responses.

Laugh with — not at.

The role of family and friends

There is an old saying that you can choose your friends but you can't choose your family. While this may apply in some families under certain circumstances, it is interesting to see what happens when the chips are down. As the news of the diagnosis of breast cancer spreads through the family, in-fighting, bickering, old disputes, and differences are suddenly all forgotten as everyone rallies to face the common enemy — cancer — which is threatening a family member and indirectly threatening them.

Suddenly people are doing here, helping there, buying this, bringing that, visiting and chatting, interested in helping. Why is it that we only really respond to one another when there is a risk factor involved? Why do we allow so many situations to occur where we end up saying 'If only ... '? Why do we only appreciate something when we feel we may lose it, or sadly may already have lost it? It is as if the true value of something we care about becomes apparent when our priorities are questioned. Renewing old relationships, improving previous friendships, giving new values to things that we nearly lost through lack of trying a little harder — all these are positive aspects of facing cancer in our lives. They are the hidden bonuses in the process. Look out for them and make full use of them.

Friends fall into many categories and can be supportive in many ways: as confidant(e)s with whom personal and private matters can be intimately discussed; as companions who are affectionate, reliable, and who usually cheer you up; as a familiar clique where you know you are fully accepted; or as cronies who are attached, devoted, faithful, and loyal to you. Some of us are fortunate enough to have friends of long-standing, who know and understand us and who have travelled a long way with us. Some may already have shared other troubles with us; they understand us and what makes us tick. Other friendships may be of shorter duration, but may still be just as genuine, loyal, and supportive. Call on friends: let them spoil you, let them do little things for you, let them share with you some of your fear, anger, and worry. They are there for you, but you must also be there for them. Don't shut them out; don't exclude them. In allowing them to help you, the bonds of friendship can be strengthened further to help with trying times ahead.

Let family and friends help.

66 *Through this experience family and friends have expressed emotions and feelings that they normally would not have. It was touching to know how special they thought I was and how much they loved me.* **Jenny** 99

The role of doctors

There is no doctor as valuable as a good general practitioner who knows you, your personal life, your circumstances, your strengths, your weaknesses, and your ability to cope with certain decisions and situations. A comfortable, honest, friendly relationship with your doctor is something which will be of tremendous help during the counselling, decision-making, and adapting stages of breast cancer. His or her explanation, support, and empathy can help to alleviate or prevent many problems which may arise. Giving honest, qualified answers to your many probing questions (thus allowing for full understanding and awareness of possibilities and prospects) is as invaluable as the guidance and suggestions your doctor can also provide.

Unfortunately (or fortunately, depending on how you look at it) you will also need to be seen by someone who is a stranger to you — the surgeon. You will usually not know him, and you will be referred by your general practitioner. If you see a doctor at a state hospital, she will also refer you to the surgical department for planning the form, type, and time of surgery. This means getting to know someone completely new to you who is going to guide, advise, and inform you about a bewildering choice of courses of action. The choice is also pretty final, as there is usually very little room for manoeuvring once a certain direction has been chosen as regards lumpectomy or modified mastectomy. You may of course meet the surgeon for the first time while still at that scary stage of needing a lump biopsied and awaiting the diagnosis.

Remember the shopping list of questions for your doctor? The same applies for your surgeon: write down things that you want clarified and get answers when next you see him. Do not be afraid to ask, and do not consider any question that worries you too trivial. Remember, the unasked questions may remain unanswered. It is much better to ask rather than worry— often unnecessarily — about questions to which explanatory answers can go a long way to alleviating fears.

Other doctors you may come into contact with are the radiologist (through mammography), the ultrasonographer (through sonography), and the oncologist (for chemotherapy). They are all experts in their fields and are generally helpful, friendly, and pleased to answer questions and keep you informed about what the procedures or treatment entails. Do not feel anxious about asking questions or expressing any worries you have concerning any of the procedures being done.

Doctors are ordinary human beings who through specialized training and experience are competent to provide certain services using specific skills and knowledge. This does not mean that on graduating they all received a sparkling new, open, friendly personality with good communication skills as well. Like everyone they have their strengths, weaknesses, and particular personalities which you must relate to. If you find there is a strong personality clash between you and the surgeon or oncologist you have been referred to, if you are not comfortable, or if you do not have complete trust in him or her, then rather change doctors. Such a feeling of trust is usually not determined by skills or ability, but by that ill-defined interpersonal relationship that is so important between people and which often manifests as a spontaneous like or dislike on meeting for the first time.

The role of religion

Faith cannot be measured by any rational means. It has no beginning, middle, or end; it just is. It is a force that knows no bounds, that does not bow down or give way to any threat, that can overcome all logical obstacles, and that has an unlimited power to provide support in difficult circumstances. Faith is a belief that defies scientific definition, let alone understanding. It is an inner strength, a constant travelling companion through all the trials and tribulations of life. It is closely entwined with our wondrous creation and living; it is part of our awareness of the complexities and magnitude of life and death. It gives hope to the hopeless, meaning to the depressed, and direction to the lost.

For those who have faith during this trying time, their belief in God can continue to grow and can be a tremendous source of strength and support. Your God is a friend who will always be there for you through these frightening and stressful experiences; one who never has a closed door or an 'Out to lunch' sign — He is on call 24 hours a day, 365 days a year.

For those who do not have their faith to rely on, this can be a very important time to open yourself up to it. Human nature is such that when we find ourselves under siege, when we seem to have lost control and events are overtaking us, we turn much more readily to religion. What fair-weather travellers many of us are: when all is well, we have no interest in matters of faith, but when the tables turn and life is not going so well, we are suddenly ready to ask for forgiveness and help.

Cancer can act as the catalyst for you to re-introduce yourself to faith. It can help and strengthen you in so many ways.

Faith is a small word for an enormous force.

Your role: Mind, body, and attitude

This has been quite fully covered previously, so a brief synopsis only is given here.

Become — and stay — physical. Improve both body and mind. Establish new goals and priorities in life. Remember that fortune is stable in one thing — she does not like faint hearts. The hour of greatest tiredness is just before the goal is reached, so persevere, do not give up. Do not start something and say, 'Oh what the heck, what's the use?' In many ways at this time of your life indecision is a very near relative to unhappiness. So decide on a course or direction and go for it. Do not let hope escape: for those who hope not, the unhoped-for will never come. Look on this stage as the beginning of the rest of your life. You have been given a reprieve, another chance; do not let it go to waste through worry and negative attitudes. Look on it as a half-full bottle rather than a half-empty one. The part of life that is over, including its fears, sacrifices, and suffering, is done with and cannot be changed. You cannot live in Fairyland and say, 'What if it had not happened to me?' What you can do is say, 'I will make the very best of the rest of my life and I will not let a day pass unappreciated or wasted.' There is so much to do: grow in your own strength and abilities; grow in your job; cultivate new interests or hobbies; practise new sports or activities; renew and strengthen old friendships; travel more; explore your own town, city, gardens, parks, museums, and theatres; appreciate the wonders and splendours of nature. Don't say, 'Why I can't', but say, 'Why I should', and do something about it. Life can become more exciting and much more meaningful when it is threatened. It is as if you have a new set of weights, measures, and scales with which to re-assess the value of your everyday living.

You are never too old to grow.

66 *I often quote a little saying — I have no idea of the origin, but it is very wise: "If it were not for the rocks in its bed, the stream would have no song."* **Jenny** 99

The role of natural healing

Here I am alluding to all forms of healing other than allopathic (conventional) medicine. Any doctor worthy of respect will accept that there are different ways of achieving certain ends; that there is more than one way of getting better; and that belief in a particular method is an important ingredient for success. I am happy to accept that additional help and support can be achieved through natural healing methods.

I would, however, be failing totally in my duty to you if I ever advocated that natural healing be allowed to replace the scientifically proven methods of surgery, radiotherapy, chemotherapy, and hormone therapy. That would be inviting a tragedy, and I cannot under any circumstances recommend that you discontinue the proven treatment protocols and opt for natural healing on its own.

However, if you do feel strongly about it, then natural treatment as an extra support can be arranged. This will need to be discussed fully with your doctor in case of possible interactions or side-effects. Additional vitamins, trace elements, and healthy, nutritional eating are clearly of benefit. The use of non-toxic herbal mixtures is also fine. Mixtures with potential side-effects should not, however, be taken without consultation to establish when and how they can safely be used. If you are in any doubt, discuss the preparations with your doctor first.

Include natural healing
but do not exclude conventional medicine.

Chapter 12

Follow-up and further care

Once treatment is complete

It all happened so quickly: first there was the lump; then the worry; then the biopsy; then the worry; then the choice between lumpectomy or mastectomy; then the surgery; then the physiotherapy; then perhaps also the radiation or chemotherapy; and then still the worry.

When you have been cured of cancer there remains an irrepressible, niggling worry that pops up with any new symptom you have. That back-ache that is perhaps more painful than usual after gardening — is it a secondary? These headaches you are having — what do they really mean? Am I losing weight too easily? I know I had arthritis before, but were my joints as sore as this? And so it goes on and on. As time passes and the false alarms continue, you will begin to realize that they are all part of normal living and not part of more cancer. Often establishing this and getting further reassurance may require further tests.

No matter how logical, organized, or sensible you are about the whole question of breast cancer, and even if you feel that you 'have it all in perspective', the worried times are never going to be completely over. Coping with breast cancer is a lifetime problem. Regular follow-up with your doctor is important. Depending on the staging and type of cancer that you had, follow-up will take different forms, with further tests or scans being indicated under certain conditions. In most cases further tests and follow-up will just be safety precautions which are being taken to detect as early as possible any recurrence which may occur and then to plan the course of action that needs to be taken.

It may be worth looking again at why early detection of cancer in the first place is so important, and how it improves your chances. As regards the likelihood of recurrence of the same cancer, after a five-year disease-free period you will be considered cured and free of that specific cancer, but recurrences may rarely occur as long as fifteen years after the primary lesion was removed.

Why follow-up is so important

While the nature and forms of the different breast cancers are becoming better understood, there is no full understanding of what to expect from cancer *in situ*. There is an overall recurrence rate of around 7% for cancer in the other breast within five to ten years of the first cancer. Some women are so worried about a recurrence that they opt for a prophylactic mastectomy, but some interesting and in some ways reassuring facts arise: when careful histology is done on the symptom-free breast tissue (removed prophylactically), up to a third of patients will have one or more sites of cancer *in situ,* and yet only 7% will have developed a progressive cancer in the next ten years.

What is even more interesting and confusing is that cancer *in situ* occurring within the duct (ductal carcinoma) is much more likely to become invasive then cancer *in situ* occurring with the lobule (lobular carcinoma). Other histological features are also indications that tumours have different 'personalities': some are very placid and remain unobtrusive, while others are much more aggressive and uncontrolled. The personality of the tumour bears no relation to the personality of the patient! But it does govern its behaviour, and this can affect the outlook. So regular follow-up is essential.

Stage	Breast-cancer type	Five-year survival rate %
0	Cancer *in situ*	98–100
1	Local invasive cancer, glands negative (clear)	90
2	Local invasive cancer with 1–3 glands involved	70–80
3	Spread to glands with more than 4 glands involved	50–60
4	Distant spread to other organs, bones, etc.	10
	Local very advanced cancer	20

Table 12.1 *Breast cancer five-year survival rates*

What is also quite clear is that the body's defence mechanisms are effective in controlling or destroying the majority of *in situ* carcinoma.

Follow-up routine

This routine is essential for all women who have had breast cancer:
- self-examination must be done carefully and diligently on a monthly basis;
- biannual breast examination by your doctor;
- annual mammography of the remaining breast, or of both breasts in the event of a lumpectomy; and
- awareness of increased risk and therefore of the need to be more careful. Such awareness becomes part of your life but must not be allowed to govern it.

What if all the treatment does not work?

This is where we come to the scary and sobering reality of cancer of the breast. It is by far the commonest cancer in women, and worldwide over a million women will be diagnosed annually. About one third of these women will die within ten years of its diagnosis. Most of them will have been stage III or IV at diagnosis, but some (much fewer) will be from stages I and II. That is why this book has concentrated on the crucial importance of early detection and active, aggressive management. Sadly, however, there are no absolute guarantees of cure even with early detection. Does one ever 'win' with cancer? The answer is yes, but always at a cost. There are no easy victories; there is always a price to pay.

How do you 'win'?

1 You may win totally with 'minimal' trauma (damage) from the battle. You may overcome the mastectomy and/or lumpectomy, have your radiation (in the case of a lumpectomy), require no chemotherapy, have your reconstruction done without major problems regarding your femininity and body image, and return to your previous life wiser, thankful, and with new goals and priorities.
2 You may still win, as in (1), but only after paying the additional price of having chemotherapy, loss of hair, feeling nauseous,

and having to delay reconstructive surgery for at least six months. But in the end you are cured, reconstruction — if so desired — can be done, and you continue with life as in (1).

3   You may still win, as with (1) and (2), but may require further treatment for a local recurrence which will need further surgery and/or radiation and/or chemotherapy. You are cured after all this, but having travelled a much tougher road to reach the goal of being healed.

4   Or you may win as in (1), (2), or (3), but you will be amongst the 7% who will get a second cancer in the other breast. 'Good news' (if there is such a thing under the circumstances) is that your outlook remains excellent if the second cancer is found early. This is likely to be the case, because you will have been followed up carefully with regular breast examinations, annual mammograms, and so on.

5   Or you may not win. There is no way I can alter, hide, or diminish the seriousness of this situation, when distant metastasis (spread) has occurred and the disease is in its stage 4 phase. Even then the situation is not totally hopeless, as much can still be done with different chemotherapy and hormone regimes of treatment. They can cause regression (retreat) of the cancer which can last for long periods (years). The next best that can be achieved is that the cancer can be held in check and its progression stopped for reasonably long periods of time. At very least the tumours' progression is slowed but not stopped, and this is usually for shorter periods — months rather than years. In addition there are many other aspects of healing which cannot be scientifically measured or documented in a laboratory. These include the power of religion, the power and complexity of the mind and the will to live, the power of self-healing through the body's own defences, and finally the power of other remedies and modalities of natural healing. The one rule in this situation is that no rule is applicable in every case!

Facing the prospect of dying

This is such a personal and intimate period of individual adjustment that in many ways it is presumptuous of me even to offer advice or solace. How can one truly understand if you have not had to face such a reality yourself; one where the waves of turmoil and tragedy batter at the strongest defences you can erect? There have, however, been many situations in my medical life where I have seen different reactions, and different coping strategies used, whether while adjusting to

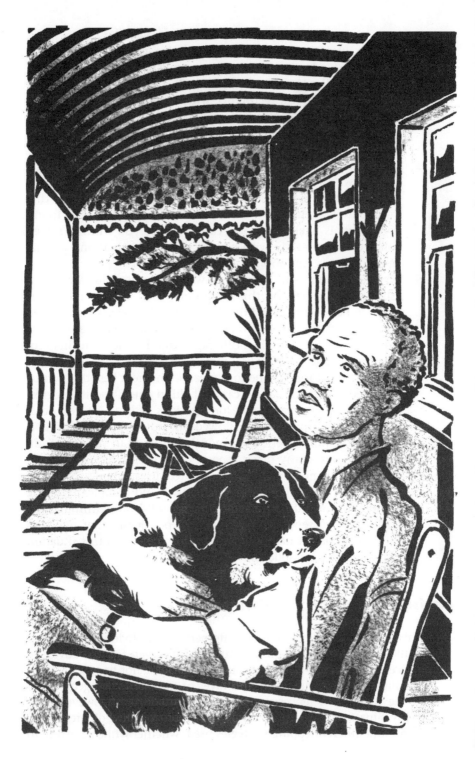

the loss of a child or an adult loved-one or to the prospect of death.

- For some people, death itself is not as frightening as the *process* of dying. What is feared most is the pain, suffering, and loss of dignity.
- Many are doubtful about the existence of a life-after-death. Death is therefore seen as an absolute end, a nothingness that is hard to imagine, which makes the prospect of dying particularly hard to come to terms with.
- Even for people who have a strong belief in some form of after-life, anticipating the transition may cause a lot of apprehension.
- Some feel 'cheated' by their approaching end; they cannot stop feeling, 'Why did this happen to *me*?'. They may fight on to the last, refusing to acknowledge that they are very close to dying.
- Others isolate themselves and withdraw, becoming almost impossible to approach. Attempts to comfort them may be met with a cold-shouldered reproach.
- Some people seem to 'resign themselves' to dying, and wait passively, with little resistance or complaint.
- Others keep themselves busy organizing everything they can to assist family and friends. They show an often-cheerful determination to enjoy the last days of earthly life to the full, sharing love and closeness with family and friends. Such people often accept death calmly and philosophically, particularly if they have a strong inner faith.

Whatever your response if you are faced with death from cancer, remember that there are many people who care and who can help by sharing your burden: not only family and friends to support you, but also doctors and nurses who can ensure that you do not suffer indignity or unbearable pain. Let others help you. Do not try to bear it alone.

There is no single strategy that can possibly work for everyone, but here are a few common denominators that can form a basis on which you can build your own coping strategy.

General principles

The old Chinese saying 'If you help someone up a hundred steps they will need your help most on the last one' is very appropriate when you are terminally ill. Do not try to face the prospect alone: the last step *is* the one when you will be most in need of help and support.

There are always sources of help — more so in some situations than in others, but never such that there are none at all. They can be family, friends, doctors, oncologists, specialized nurses, support groups (for example, prayer groups or women who have had breast cancer), psychologists and psychiatrists, ministers of religion, and the hospice movement (including home visiting). The degree and extent of involvement of these help-sources will vary depending on the stage of the disease and the physical and emotional needs of the individual. If there is a good support infrastructure of family and friends, with guidance from a wide range of professionals, it is often a therapeutic balm for many of the emotional ills and fears being experienced.

Cancer is an unpredictable disease, and while it usually follows certain rules, it does not do so in all cases. You are an individual with a disease that may be following its own set of rules. Even with advanced cancer, response to therapy can be very positive, with control of pain and regression being achieved, so it is best not to plan too far ahead or consider death as inevitable. While we must consider the tomorrows of our life, a good motto to bear in mind in this situation is, 'Give me today and tomorrow will take care of itself'. Go step by step, day by day, facing problems only if and when they arise. Many may not arise at all, and others when faced squarely may not be as bad or difficult as you originally imagined.

There are recognized phases which one goes through under these 'coming-to-grips-with-your-disease' circumstances. First, there is usually the phase of denial: 'Oh no, it cannot be true. It cannot happen to me.' This often changes to one of anger: 'Why me? What have I done to deserve this? It's so damn unfair.' Thereafter there is the process of bargaining: 'If I do this or do that, then I will have longer to live.' And finally you come to the stage of accepting the reality of the situation. Coming to terms with dying is therefore an ongoing process, never static, and it takes time. Loved-ones and friends must be aware of possible reactions during these phases, and must see such reactions in perspective. The Chinese often have a 'screaming tree' in their back yard. Such a tree (often a mulberry) becomes the object on which anger, frustration, fear, and anguish is vented: the tree is shouted at, screamed at, and verbally abused as an emotional outlet-valve. So, too, anger, frustration, or fear may be 'taken out' on a loved-one or friend, who may be very hurt or perplexed by this unwarranted reaction. They may then withdraw their support, in ignorance. If this should happen, it is up to both of you to put matters straight once the 'eruption' has settled down and your anger or fears can be discussed more rationally. They must see that they served the important function and role of a 'screaming tree'. This may be difficult to understand, and requires a mature, balanced attitude.

What is feared most?

Many patients are more frightened of pain than of actually dying. Pain need never become unbearable. There are many strategies that can be used in its control. With some cancers, hormonal therapy can be very effective in pain-control. Individual secondaries which are causing a particular problem can be shrunk with local radiation and thereby pain is reduced. There are also many forms of analgesics (pain-killers) which can be used. They come in varying strengths and lengths of action (effect). With modern drugs you do not have to be in a 'woozy' (sleepy, out-of-contact) state of mind. Clarity of thought and full awareness of your environment is usually possible. Another group of drugs which is helpful is the anti-inflammatories. These may be used as additional supportive therapy.

Pain-control is essential, and you must insist upon as much as is required in your particular case. It is not necessary to have to suffer unbearable pain at any stage. Yes, there will be times when the degree of discomfort will be extreme, but it can and must be brought under control. Make your doctor aware of your needs and wishes. Unfortunately some doctors are still relatively conservative as regards pain-control, and you may need to 'educate' them in this regard. There are also doctors who specialize in pain-control, and it may be worth having a discussion with such a specialist as to what can and should be done. The hospice movement personnel, due to their experience, are usually excellent in this regard, and their aim is to relieve pain and suffering as much as is humanly possible.

The power of your mind

Once again, some of the responsibility falls on you, as you yourself are an important part of the coping strategy with regard to pain or discomfort. You must remain strong-willed and not crumble in the face of discomfort. You must work at fortitude and you must strengthen your resolve to do so. You are aiming for a delicate balance between accepting the situation but not giving in to it. You can take pride in your coping strategies; you can gain in inner strength as you maintain your position of control. Do not give up before the approaching final battle is fought. But do not attempt to fight it alone. Around you are many people who are sympathetic to your needs. Sympathy has been defined as the power of knowing without being told. This may be true sometimes, but at times it will be necessary for you to express your needs to those who are anxious to help. Open the door to their silent knocking — they will often be ill-at-ease and may avoid the issue of cancer to such an extent that you have to take the initiative in talking about it.

Speaking is not always necessary: sometimes the mere physical presence of a loved-one can be very reassuring, and understanding silence can be as good as, if not better than, conversation. Actions can often say more than words, so support can take many forms. Just being with you as you read a book, or holding your hand as you drift off to sleep can be invaluable companionship.

Honesty and discussion

The father of one of our friends had a leg amputated because of a bone cancer. On meeting him for the first time, most people would look everywhere but at the remaining stump, would discuss everything but what had happened to his leg, and would totally avoid any reference to any aspect of cancer, amputation, pain, or his feelings and fears. Our young twin daughters, with the inquisitive honesty of children, walked straight up to him, took one look at the stump as he sat in the wheelchair and said, 'Where has your leg gone? Is it sore? Will you get another one? Can you walk with only one leg?' and so on. When told that the leg was cut off by a doctor because there was something wrong inside it, the next questions were: 'Why? When? How?', and so on it went in this honest enquiring theme. The old man was eventually chuckling to himself as he tried to answer all the forthright and honest questions.

He remarked to us afterwards what a delightful experience it had been to be asked direct questions, to have issues confronted and not studiously avoided or ignored, and to be able to look someone in the eye and not merely in the face, as they avoided eye contact with him. So what is the lesson? The lesson is that we should all be much more like children — without of course being unintentionally 'cruel' as children sometimes are through not knowing when to stop pursuing an issue. Such insight and finer judgement only comes with experience in life, but we can certainly learn a lot from children as regards candour and honesty.

We should discuss things openly rather than pretending that they do not exist. Many people do not know how to do this; they will not enter into an area where they feel uncomfortable, awkward, and ill-at-ease. However, if you make the first move and encourage them ever so slightly to enter that 'forbidding area', they will gain in confidence, and before you know where you are, hidden fears need be hidden no more. You all gain — the 'supporters' and the patient. With subsequent developments in the disease process and with further progression there is then no 'barrier of silence', no awkwardness to overcome, and new problems or fears can be dealt with in a forthright and constructive manner.

Encourage those who want to help to do so. In many ways you are the conductor of the Orchestra of Support, and you can therefore decide on the form, nature, and length of the support melody you currently wish to hear: while many will still feel it is just too private to share, and they do not know how to go about it, I would encourage you to share your fears with a loved-one, dear friend, your doctor, or minister of religion. Once you overcome the fence of isolation you have erected around your own inner thoughts and fears, discussion becomes easier. You may even require a professional counsellor to help with this process of facilitating discussion.

Specific coping strategies

These are varied and personal, depending on what you find most helps your own specific needs. What works for some may not work for others. When faced with the prospect of dying, your dependence on loved-ones, family, friends, your religion and the ministers of that religion, your doctor and health-care workers will vary tremendously with your emotional needs and the stage of your disease.

One important denominator is common to all coping strategies: sharing your fears and worries with someone is essential. The other very important ingredient in the whole process is of course yourself. Never underestimate your own ability and strength of purpose: take pride in them, take pride in coping, believe in yourself and that you can do it.

> 66 *I look on the experience as a positive one. I have made friends and helped people I would never normally have met, and the reward of tears being replaced by brave smiles has for me been a special experience in itself.* **Jenny** 99

> 66 *With each new symptom or ache I still dread that it signals the return of cancer. I suppose this is something I am just going to have to live with.* **Jenny** 99

Appendix I

The Cancer Association of South Africa
Toll free number: 0800 22 6622 (8.30 – 12.30)

National Office
Box 2000
Johannesburg
2000
(011) 403 2825

Eastern Cape
Box 7192
Port Elizabeth
6055

Port Elizabeth
(041) 35 1212

Uitenhage
(0422) 992 6767

East London
(0431) 2 6081

OFS & Northern Cape
Box 1686
Bloemfontein
9300

Bloemfontein
(051) 47 7534

Kimberley
(0531) 81 2968

Kroonstad
(01411) 5 1408

Welkom
(0171) 3 2112

Northern Transvaal
Box 275
Pretoria
0001

Pretoria
(012) 329 3036

Nelspruit
(01311) 5 2435/6

Pietersburg
(01521) 91 1298/9

Rustenburg
(0142) 2 8980

Witbank
(0135) 5420/2211

Southern Transvaal
Box 32979
Braamfontein
2017

Johannesburg
(011) 403 3300

Ermelo
(01341) 5893/4

Kempton Park
(011) 393 1141/2

Klerksdorp
(018) 2 9894

Roodepoort
(011) 766 2909

Secunda
(01363) 4 1103

Springs
(011) 815 2342

Vereeniging
(016) 22 4897

Natal
Box 17173
Congella
4013

Durban
(031) 25 9525

Ladysmith
(0361) 2 2104

Pietermaritzburg
(0331) 42 9837

South Coast
(0323) 2 2041

Western Cape
Box 186
Rondebosch
7700

Cape Town
(021) 689 5347

Langa
(021) 648 1841/2

Paarl
(02211) 2 6045

Oudtshoorn
(0443) 22 2724

George
(0441) 74 4824

Worcester
(0231) 2 7058

Goodwood
(021) 592 3073/4/6

Fundraising number:
01 10000 2000 0
Reg. no: 05/03720/08

Appendix II

Hospice Association of Southern Africa

P O Box 602, Durbanville
7550
Tel: (021) 448 7624
Fax: (021) 47 4379
Contact: National Secretary, Peter Buckland

Full members:

Highway Hospice
P O Box 28, Westville
3630
Tel: (031) 28 6110
Fax: (031) 28 2945
Contact: Sr Greta Schoeman

St Francis Hospice
P O Box 12128, Centrahil
6006
Tel: (041) 30 7070
Fax: (041) 30 1279
Contact: Sr Lesley Lawson

St Luke's Hospice
P O Box 59, Kenilworth
7745
Tel: (021) 797 5335
Fax: (021) 761 0130
Contact: Sr Hilary Strickland

Associate members:

Bloemfontein Hospice
P O Box 28391, Danhof
9310
Tel: (051) 47 7281
Contact: Sr Joan Marston

Edendale Hospice Association
Private Bag 9099,
Pietermaritzburg
3200
Tel: (0331) 954 1154
Fax: (0331) 95 4031
Contact: Sr Mary Moleko

Goldfields Hospice
P O Box 1556, Welkom
9460
Tel: (0171) 353 2152
Fax: (0171) 353 4197
Contact: Mrs Val Bekker

Grahamstown Hospice Service
P O Box 664, Grahamstown
6140
Tel: (0461) 2 9661
Contact: Mrs Robin Kent

Helderberg Hospice
P O Box 1640, Somerset West
7130
Tel: (024) 852 4608
Contact: Sr Pat Pigeon

Hospice Association of the East Rand
P O Box 13454, Northmead
1511
Tel: (011) 422 1531
Fax: (011) 54 4785
Contact: Sr Pet Birchall

Hospice Association of Pretoria
P O Box 90554, Garsfontein
0042
Tel: (012) 47 4909
Fax: (012) 348 5414
Contact: Sr Sheila Lahou

Hospice in the West
P O Box 1694, Krugersdorp
1740
Tel: (011) 953 4863
Fax: (011) 953 4738
Contact:
Mrs Marisa Wolheim

Hospice Western Transvaal
P O Box 2993, Klerksdorp
2570
Tel: (018) 484 3374
Contact: Mrs Audrey Rudd

Howick Hospice
P O Box 819, Howick
3290
Tel: (0332) 30 5257
Contact: Mrs Shirley Cloete

Knysna/Sedgefield Hospice
P O Box 1348, Knysna
6570
Tel: (0445) 2 4637
Contact: Sr Fiona Simpson

Lighthouse Hospice
P O Box 144, Umkomaas
4170
Tel: (0323) 3 1032
Contact: Mrs Natalie Sinclair

Pietermaritzburg Hopsice
P O Box, 11340, Dorpspruit
3206
Tel: (0331) 44 1560
Fax: (0331) 94 0504
Contact: Mrs Clare Wylie

South Coast Hospice
P O Box 504, Port Shepstone
4240
Tel: (0391) 2 3031
Fax: (c/o Hudson & Naude)
   (0391) 82 4694
Contact: Sr Kath Defilippi

Wide Horizons Hospice Vaal Triangle
P O Box 2911, Vereeniging
1930
Tel: (016) 28 1410
Fax: (016) 63 1329
Contact: Dr Isak Steyl

Affiliate members
Regional associations:

Hospice Association of Natal
P O Box 819, Howick
3290
Tel: (031) 28 6110
Contact: Sr Karen Hinton

Associations in service:

Chatsworth Hospice
RK Khan Hospital
Private Bag X004,
Chatsworth
4030

Estcourt Hospice
P O Box 75, Estcourt
3310
Tel: (0363) 33 5634
Contact: Eileen Portsmouth
(Secretary)

Hospice Association of Kimberley
c/o P O Box 1596, Kimberley
8300
Tel: (0531) 2 4472
Contact: Mrs Gus Williamson

Hospice Association of the Witwatersrand
P O Box 87600, Houghton
2041
Tel: (011) 483 1068 or 3256
Fax: (011) 728 3104
Contact: Sr Janet Frohlich

Parys Hospice
97 Schilbach Street, Parys
9585
Contact: Mr P F van Zijl

St Bernard's Hospice
44 St Mark's Road, East
London
5201
Tel: (0431) 2 3575
Contact: Dr Betty Bennett

Stellenbosch Hopsice
P O Box 3161, Coetzenburg
7602
Tel: (02231) 83 2701
Contact: Sr Libby Reinecke

Swaziland Hospice at Home
P O Box 23, Matsapha
Swaziland
Tel: (w) (09268) 5 5402
     (h) (09268) 8 5521

Vryheid Hospice
P O Box 210, Vryheid
3100
Tel: (0381) 80 9888
Contact: Sr Zilla Foster.
Tel: (0381) 3369
Mrs Zelda France-Brotherton.
Tel: (0381) 4988

Zululand Hospice
P O Box 289, Empangeni
3880
Contact: Willi Miller

Honorary member

Mr Brian Agar
P O Box 35
Durban
4000

Mailing list

Ramotswa Hospice at Home
P O Box 6 Ramotswa Village
Botswana
Tel: (09267) 39 0212
Contact: Sr Christa Kiebel-
stein

Franschhoek Voluntary Home Nursing and Hospice Service
P O Box 257, Franschhoek
7690
Tel: (02212) 2527
Contact: Mrs Versveld

Island Hospice
P O Box 8246, Causeway,
Harare
Zimbabwe
Tel: (09263 4) 79 1605
Contact: Dave McElavine

Kroonstad Hospice
P O Box 1265, Kroonstad
9500
Tel: (h) (01411) 5104
    (w) (01411) 5511
Contact: Dr J S van der Poel

Mahyeno Mission
P O Box 503, Dundee
3000
Tel: (0341) 2 4445

Eshowe Hospice
P O Box 32, Unkwaleni
3816
Contact: Lorraine du Plessis

Paarl Hospice
P O Box 6130, Main Street,
Paarl
7622
Tel: (02211) 2 4060 (9 <197>
12 noon, Tuesdays only)
Fax: (02211) 2 7133 (mark
'for attention Paarl Hospice')
Contact: Dr M Snyman

Rietvlei Hospital (Home Care Group)
P O Staffords Post, Via Hard-
ing
4680
Contact: Mrs Janice Whit-
taker

Tzaneen Care Group
P O Box 4, Ofcolaco
0854
Contact: Mrs H M Geddes

Nairobi Hospice
P O Box 74818, Nairobi
Kenya
Tel: (09254 2) 72 2212

Kangwane College of Nursing
Private Bag X1005,
Kabokweni
1245
Tel: (01316) 96 0244/5

Glossary

This is a list of technical and medical words used in this book to describe aspects of breast lumps, breast cancer, and its treatment. Also included are some additional terms that you may hear doctors use during the investigation and management of your breast problem.

Abscess
A painful, boil-like infection in the breast

Adenoma
Non-cancerous growth in glandular body tissue

Adenocarcinoma
A cancer of glandular tissue

Adjuvant
Means back-up or additional. Word used when talking about further treatments for cancer, e.g., chemotherapy

Alopecia
Loss of hair, particularly on the head

Amenorrhoea
The absence of periods

Antibody
Produced as part of the immune system's response to protect the body from disease, especially bacterial and viral infection

Antigen
Foreign stimulus for antibody production

Antineoplastic
Another term for cytotoxic and chemotherapeutic agents

Areola
The circular darker/pinker area of skin surrounding the nipple

Arteries
Vessels (high pressure) which carry the blood from the heart to all parts of the body

Aspiration
Withdrawing fluid or cells from a cyst or body tissue using a needle attached to a syringe

Axilla
Armpit

Bacteria
Micro-organisms found in plants, animals, and humans. May be beneficial, safe, or dangerous (disease-causing)

Benign tumour
Non-cancerous growth which does not invade other tissue or spread to other sites in the body by blood and lymph

Biopsy
Removal of a small amount of breast tissue which is then studied under a microscope to determine its character

Capillary
Minute blood vessels at the ends of arteries supplying blood to body tissues

Carcinogen
A substance which can cause cancerous changes to occur in cells

Carcinoma
A cancerous growth of epithelial cells. These cells line the body's external and internal surfaces, such as the skin, large intestine, lungs, stomach, cervix, and breast

(ducts and channels). Carcinomas invade surrounding tissue and may spread through the body to other sites by blood and lymph

Carcinoma *in situ*
A cancerous growth which has not yet invaded surrounding tissue. It occurs in the milk ducts and breast lobules

Cardiovascular system
The network of blood vessels (which includes veins, arteries, and capillaries) and the heart, which pumps blood throughout the body

Cell differentiation
The process whereby cells of a common origin maintain special functions and characteristics. Cancer cells often lose this ability

Chemotherapy
Treatment by one or more drugs which are capable of destroying cancer cells and other rapidly reproducing cells such as hair and marrow

Chronic
Persistent or long-lasting

Circumscribed carcinoma
A well-defined cancer with a capsule-like outer layer. Usually slow-growing carcinoma

Clinical trials
Carefully organized tests which aim to assess the effectiveness of particular forms of treatment for a disease

Consultant
Senior doctor specializing in a particular area of medicine. Also called a specialist

Corticosteroids
Hormones with strong anti-inflammatory and anti-cancer (in some cases) activity. Have many side-effects

Cyst
Sack filled with fluid

Cytology
Study of cells' character through staining and histology

Cytoplasm
Substance comprising the main part of a cell within the cell wall. Other cellular components are found within it

Cytotoxic drugs
Drugs which damage and destroy cancer cells

Differentiation
See cell differentiation

DNA
Genetic blueprint of the species in the nucleus of a cell (DNA stands for deoxyribonucleic acid)

Duct
A tube-like channel carrying fluid, such as the milk ducts in the breast

Duct ectasia
Enlargement and hardening of a diseased duct accompanied by discharge from the nipple

Dysplasia
Abnormal cell features used to describe non-cancerous or pre-cancerous cell changes

Endocrine system
Glands and their hormones that circulate in the body and have an effect on organs and tissues

Environment
The different things in our lives which effect us socially, physically, and personally, e.g., pollution, diet, housing, income, weather.

Enzyme
Protein produced in a cell which facilitates cell function

Epithelium
Sheet of cells that lines tubes, cavities, and surfaces in the body. Most cancers originate from epithelial cells

Excision
Removal of tissue through surgery

Fat necrosis
Death of fat cells, which can be the cause of a lump in the breast

Fibroadenoma
Non-cancerous growth of fibrous and glandular tissue. Fibroadenosis is a more generalized spread of this condition. A lactational adenoma is a fibroadenoma which develops during pregnancy

Fibrocystic disease
Non-cancerous condition producing cysts and fibrous tissue in the breast

Fibrous tissue
Tissue consisting of fibres, sometimes increased as a response to disease or scar tissue

Fibrosis
Collection of fibrous tissue

Frozen section
Biopsy performed and studied while patient is under a general anaesthetic. The tissue sample is rapidly frozen to enable speedy cutting and histology to be done

Gene
A section of DNA which contains the information coding for an inherited characteristic, such as eye colour

Glands
Structures in the body producing hormones which affect different parts of the body, e.g., the ovaries

Histology
Study of body tissue using a microscope and staining of cells

Hormone
Chemical message which produces changes in the behaviour of specific cells

Hormone-replacement therapy (HRT)
Hormonal treatment used to replace oestrogen during and after the menopause

Hospice
Place providing special care for those who are dying

Hyperplasia
Increased cell production which is not cancerous

Hysterectomy
Surgical removal of the womb and/or ovaries

Immune system
Body's system for detection of and protection from many forms of disease, including cancer

Immunotherapy
Treatment which aims to improve the efficiency of the immune system

Implant (breast)
Artificial breast-form, usually made of silicone placed beneath the skin or chest muscle following a mastectomy

Inflammatory breast cancer
Painful but rare cancer causing generalized inflammation of the breast

Informed consent
Fully understanding the implications of a procedure, the alternatives, and possible risks before consenting to it being done

In situ
Cancer which has not yet invaded surrounding tissue (Latin for 'in place')

Intracystic
Within a cyst

Intraductal cancer
Cancer which starts in the milk ducts

Intraductal papilloma
See papilloma

Invasive cancer
Cancer which has spread into surrounding tissue

Ionizing radiation
Rays of very small particles capable of damaging the genetic structure of fast-growing cells, e.g., X-rays

Keloid
Excess unattractive scar tissue

Kinetics of cell
Growing and multiplying characteristics of a cell

Lactation
Milk production in the breast for feeding mammals

Lactational adenoma
See fibroadenoma

Ligament
Band of fibrous tissue strengthening the body's structure. Cooper's ligaments support the breast

Lipoma
Non-cancerous growth of fatty tissue in the breast

Lobe
Segment of an organ. A lobule is a small lobe

Lobular carcinoma in situ
Cancer of the lobules that has not invaded surrounding breast tissue

Lumpectomy
Surgical removal of a breast lump

Lymph
Fluid flowing through body tissue

Lymph nodes
Small mass of tissue in lymph channels. Lymphocytes are found in large numbers in them

Lymphatic system
Network of channels which carry lymph around the body

Lymphocytes
Cells which form an important part of the body's immune response

Lymphoedema
Accumulation of lymph causing local swelling. Can occur as a result of damage or removal of the lymph nodes in the axilla

Macrophages
Specialized cells which play an important part in the body's immune system. 'Vacuum cleaners' of the body

Malignant
Cancerous

Mammals
Animals which breast-feed their young

Mammary glands
Milk-producing glands in all mammals

Mammogram
Specialized X-ray of the breast

Mammography
Science of breast examination using X-rays

Mammoplasty
Another word for process of breast reconstruction

Mastalgia
Breast pain

Mastectomy
Surgical removal of the breast. In a radical mastectomy chest-wall muscles are removed as well

Mastitis
Term used to describe inflammation of the breast. Covers a number of breast conditions

Medullary breast cancer
Cancer which forms a well-defined lump with a capsule-like outer layer

Megadose
A very large dose of a drug or radiation

Menopause
Stage, usually between 45 and 55, when a woman stops having periods. This marks the end of a woman's reproductive life

Menstruation
Monthly periods

Metaplasia
Histological changes in cell structure which may lead to disease

Metastasis
Spread of cells from a primary cancer to form a secondary cancer elsewhere in the body. The plural is metastases

Micro-metastasis
Tiny groups of cancerous cells which spread from a primary cancer

Mitosis
Process of cell division/multiplication

Modified radical mastectomy
Surgical removal of the breast, together with the lymph nodes

Molecular genetics
Study of genetic causes and characteristics of cancer cells. May enable gene manipulation to be used therapeutically

Mortality rate
Deaths arising from a specific causative factor or group of factors. Can be expressed for sex, race, age, etc.

Mucinous breast cancer
A type of cancer in which the cancerous cells produce a mucus-like substance

Multidisciplinary team
Group of specialists with different skills giving total patient care

Necrosis
Death of tissue

Neoplasia
New and uncontrolled cell growth

Neoplasm
Tumour. Cancers are sometimes referred to as neoplasms

Non-invasive cancer
Cancer which has not spread

Nucleus
The part of a cell which contains the genetic information for identical cell growth and reproduction

Oedema
Swelling caused by fluid accumulation in body tissue

Oestrogen
Hormone produced by the ovaries which plays an important role in a woman's reproductive cycle

Oncogenes
Genes thought to be responsible for the development of certain cancers

Oncologist
A cancer specialist who may direct the overall plan of treatment for cancer

Oncology
The study and practice of treatments for all forms of cancer

Oopherectomy
Surgical removal of the ovaries but not the uterus (womb)

Osteoporosis
A condition where the bones become fragile due to mineral deficiency. Starts occurring after the menopause

Oxytocin
Hormone which stimulates milk production in breast-feeding

Paget's disease
An unusual form of breast cancer producing a skin rash of the nipple resembling eczema

Palpation
Using the hand to feel (palpate) the breast. A palpable lump is one you can feel

Papilliary breast cancer
Cancer growing in a similar way to an intraductal papilloma

Papilloma
Small non-cancerous growth like a wart. An intraductal papilloma may grow in a milk duct of the breast

Paraffin section
Setting of tissue for histology in a block of paraffin wax to enable it to be cut in thin sections

Partial mastectomy
Removal of a wedge-like portion of breast tissue including the cancer

Pathology
The biological study of disease, its causes, and its effect on the body

Pectoral muscle
Chest muscles lying immediately behind the breast

Peri-operatively
During or immediately following an operation

Phobia
An irrational, uncontrollable, excessive fear of something

Pituitary gland
Gland situated within the skull which plays an important role in the production of different hormones affecting many parts of the body

Placenta
Organ linking the unborn baby to the wall of the mother's womb. The placenta is responsible for the development and well-being of the foetus until birth

Postmenopausal
After the 'change of life'
when periods stop

Postoperatively
Period following surgery

Precancerous cells
Abnormal cells which could
develop into cancer, but do
not always

Premenopausal
Before the 'change of life'
(when periods stop)

Premenstrual
Before a period

Pre-operatively
Before surgery

Primary cancer
Original cancer from which
secondaries may spread

Progesterone
Hormone produced by the
ovaries which plays an
important role in a woman's
reproductive life. May play a
role in breast cancer

Prognosis
Working out the likely course
of a disease

Prolactin
Hormone controlling the
production of milk in a
woman who is breast-feeding

Prosthesis
A substitute or replacement
for a part of the body

Puberty
Beginning of sexual and
physical maturity

Quadrectomy
See partial mastectomy

Radiation
Rays of very small particles
which can damage cells

**Radical or classical
mastectomy**
Surgical removal of the
breast, the underlying chest
muscles, and the axillary
lymph nodes. A super-radical
mastectomy also removes the
internal chain of lymph
nodes lying beneath the
breast bone. Modified mastectomy removes only the
breast tissue and lymph
nodes in the armpit

Radiotherapy
Treatment using ionizing
radiation with the aim of
destroying cancer cells

Radium
Substance giving off ionizing
radiation

Relapse
State of recurrence of cancer
activity after it has been controlled

Remission
Period of good health following treatment of a cancer

Secondaries
Cancers in other parts of the body which develop from cells spread from a primary tumour

Segmentectomy
See partial mastectomy

Silicone implant
Artificial, inert material put into the breast by surgery to make it larger, or put under the chest muscle during reconstruction

Simulator
X-ray machine used to monitor the effects of radiotherapy on the breast and surrounding tissue

Simple mastectomy
Breast removal where the underlying chest muscles and the lymph nodes are left intact

Sinuses of the breast
Small reservoirs where milk collects during breast-feeding

Sonography
The technique of using ultrasound for diagnostic purposes. *See ultrasound*

Steroids
Hormonal drugs

Subcutaneous
Under the skin

Subcutaneous mastectomy
Removal of underlying breast tissue that leaves the skin and nipple intact

Systemic
Relating to the whole system or whole body

Tissue
General term for groups of cells in the body, usually with a particular function, e.g., the breast or the liver

Therapy
Another word for treatment, which usually covers all types of treatment or remedy

Toxic
Poisonous/damaging

Tru-cut biopsy
Using a cutting needle to obtain a specimen for histology

Tubular breast cancer
Cancer in which the cells form a tube-like pattern

Ulceration
The development of an ulcer on the skin of the breast

Ultrasound
Means of scanning body tissue and organs using sound waves to judge structure and density

Veins

Blood vessels which return blood from body tissue and lungs to the heart

Virus

Infectious agent producing disease

Vitamins

Substances essential to people's well-being which occur in many foods including vegetables and fruits

Index